ABOUT THE AUTHOR

Dr Sohère Roked, a general practitioner with a specialist interest in integrative medicine, is one of the UK's leading holistic doctors. Dr Roked has extensive knowledge of both conventional and holistic medicines and combines the two for the best possible improvement in her clients' health. A former student of the British College of Integrative Medicine, she has been taught by experts in the field from the UK, Australia and the USA. Her NHS experience made her realise what was lacking in conventional medicine, such as nutritional and lifestyle advice and how empower people to take control of their own health, and she combines her training in both to offer her patients complete health care.

I would like to dedicate this book to my mum and dad. Without their love and support and sacrifices I wouldn't be where I am today. Dad, you were my inspiration to become a doctor, and if I can only be half the doctor and person you are I will have done well.

THE
TIREDNESS
CURE

HOW TO BEAT FATIGUE AND FEEL GREAT
FOR GOOD

DR SOHÈRE ROKED

Vermilion
LONDON

1 3 5 7 9 10 8 6 4 2

Published in 2014 by Vermilion, an imprint of Ebury Publishing
Ebury Publishing is a Random House Group company

The Random House Group Limited Reg. No. 954009
Addresses for companies within the Random House Group can be found at
www.randomhouse.co.uk

A CIP catalogue record for this book is available from the British Library

The Random House Group Limited supports The Forest Stewardship Council®
(FSC®), the leading international forest-certification organisation. Our books carrying
the FSC label are printed on FSC®-certified paper. FSC is the only forest-certification
scheme supported by the leading environmental organisations, including Greenpeace.
Our paper procurement policy can be found at www.randomhouse.co.uk/environment

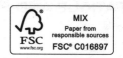

Designed and set by seagulls.net

Printed and bound by CPI Group (UK) Ltd, Croydon, CR0 4YY

ISBN 9780091955076

Copies are available at special rates for bulk orders. Contact the sales development
team on 020 7840 8487 for more information.

To buy books by your favourite authors and register for offers, visit
www.randomhouse.co.uk

CONTENTS

INTRODUCTION

Why is everyone so tired all the time? As a NHS GP this is a question I would ask myself continuously. Why are my patients so tired? Why are all my friends knackered? Hell, why was I so exhausted that I would cancel Friday-night drinks in order to lie on the sofa and fall asleep before 11 p.m.?

I remember having a conversation with a doctor I worked with in 2008 about how tired we were, while both swigging cups of coffee to keep us awake for the rest of our shift. I said quite matter-of-factly that I had come to terms with the fact that I would be tired every day for the rest of my life, and making peace with it was the best I could do. She looked at me with awe and said it was amazing I was so Zen about it. I stoically nodded, like a woman condemned to execution, accepting of my fate.

So what happened between 2008 and 2014 that made me do such a massive U-turn that I am now penning a book about how you can beat your own tiredness? As a GP, I see many patients saying they feel weak and fatigued but without any obvious medical reason. It's what I call a 'lifestyle problem', that is, it has a major impact on a person's life and well-being, but doesn't show up on conventional medical blood tests or investigations. The symptoms are certainly real, yet there's no conventional treatment for them. I've seen patients in tears as they were so physically exhausted they couldn't look after their children or get up for work in the mornings. Needless to say their quality of life was massively reduced.

It was terribly frustrating for me to see my patients in such distress without knowing how to do anything about it. So when I came across integrative medicine by chance I knew my calling was to train as an integrative medical doctor. Integrative medicine is a commonly used approach in the USA and Australia, and is even taught in the medical schools and available on the health insurance policies of those countries. Integrative medicine was not taught to me in medical school. I am sure most good doctors try to work in a holistic way by looking at a patient's lifestyle and social circumstances, but it is not specifically taught exactly how much this impacts on health and wellness. This could be to do with the way health services are funded in the UK, or perhaps to do with the current strain on the services, but it is something I hope will evolve in the future. In general, integrative medicine uses the best of Western and Eastern medicine with an evidence base and provides truly 'whole-istic' health care, looking at the whole person. I look at those niggly little symptoms that a person may be experiencing and find a way to restore the balance to the body before they accumulate and turn into an illness or disease.

As one of only ten such qualified expert doctors in the UK, I work with many private clients to help them achieve an optimum level of health. This involves a full and comprehensive consultation where I look at the individual as a 'whole', including all the factors contributing to their health and well-being. Unlike a regular GP, I'm not satisfied with the mere absence of ill health, particularly when my patients continue to feel unwell. My passion is to empower individuals to take control of their lives, to prevent illness and regenerate their health and well-being. Part of my role is to examine nutrition, fitness, stress, chemical imbalances, hormone imbalances, digestive health and toxicity in the body.

As both a NHS GP *and* a holistic doctor, I can show you how to achieve robust, enduring health through making small changes that will empower you to take control of your health and be the best *you* that you can be. I'm so confident in my programme that, if you follow it, I promise you will feel fantastic, look more youthful, get into great shape and have the energy to live your life to the full. Now who doesn't want that?

SMALL CHANGES MAKE A BIG DIFFERENCE

Is it as simple as eating well, drinking more water, managing stress and exercising? Well, in the majority of cases, yes. But I see lots of patients who do those things but still feel fatigued. In those cases we need to address other imbalances to create total health. This book will show you how. We are all busy people with lots to do, so I am going to make suggestions that fit in with your daily life and routine as much as possible.

I suggest you read the book through from start to finish and then see which chapters resonate most with you, and start with those. Alternatively, you can do the energy health check quiz in chapter 1 (see pages 12–18) and see where you score highest and start with those sections first, as this is where you need the most help. Take time to digest the information and make changes when you feel ready and able to do so. You're in this for life, not just a quick fix, so take your time.

ASSESSING YOUR CURRENT HEALTH

I have written *The Tiredness Cure* to outline a very important concept that is often forgotten:

No one should care more about your health than you do. YOU have to become the expert on you and YOU are the person responsible for your health.

Yes, *YOU!* Your GP and other health-care professionals can guide you, but ultimately, the control lies with you and the choices you make. Isn't that empowering?

The first step of the plan is to be really honest with yourself and assess where you are in your current state of energy, health and well-being. By assessing where you are now, without judgement or negativity, and stating your positive health goals, you will see more clearly where you want to go and what you want to achieve.

I would like you to answer the following questions in a notebook you can refer back to:

1. What three things would you like to change most about your health? What three things would you like to change most about your life? Are you aware of anything you currently do that could be having an impact on your health? (Think along the lines of diet, exercise, stress, smoking, alcohol, etc.)
2. What impact would changing the above have for you? How would it make you feel? How would it make things better?
3. What sort of changes could you make that would fit in with your current life?
4. How happy do you feel at the moment, and why?
5. What are your levels of stress, and why?
6. How much do you exercise? What stops you/motivates you?
7. What is your diet like? What influences this?
8. How do you think your current lifestyle will impact on your health when you are in old age?

To get the most out of this programme and become the expert on you, you have to be 100 per cent honest. Some of these questions may be hard to answer, so I'd like you to take a week to really get clear on where you are in your current state of health and well-being today, before we start to move forward. There are no right or wrong answers.

I suggest you write down the first answers you come up with and revisit them every day for 10–15 minutes and see if they need adjusting, or if you come up with new ones. At the end of the week, write down your revised answers and as the weeks go on, you will be able to see how much things are improving.

When you feel empowered you are able to take control of your health and your well-being. By taking this first step and taking responsibility, you are starting the journey to the health you've always wanted. I am committed to helping my clients achieve the best health and energy they can possibly have using new and innovative tools from integrative medicine, and I am now committed to supporting you in the same way through this book.

It's never too late to start the regeneration of your body, mind and spirit. Sometimes it seems like there's a big hill to climb that separates our current situation and the 'wellness' we want to reach. I want you to know I'm here for you and I encourage you to keep going. To be energetic and healthy is possible; just take one step at a time.

What many people don't realise is how well we are *directly* correlates with the lifestyle choices we make. For example, diet has a major impact on how we feel and our energy levels. The proportion of fruit and vegetables we eat provides energy for the body; conversely the amount of processed foods we eat zaps our energy levels. Smoking, alcohol and caffeine all zap energy too, as does stress, whereas relaxation, exercise and taking the right supplements boost our energy levels. It's also important to note that running on empty, although often commendable in our work-all-hours culture, causes a complete disruption of our natural rhythms.

HOW I CAN HELP YOU

I'm here to guide you on a new path to improve and maximise your health and this book will take you through the process step-by-step. I like takeaways, chocolate and having a good night out as much as anyone and so I am realistic and advise working by a 70/30 principle. This means implementing your new regime about five/six days a week and then you can have a few treats on the other day(s). If you're in reasonable health you will see changes within a few weeks. If you're not currently in the best shape then I would like you to try to be a bit stricter with yourself. I promise you it will be worth it.

I *know* this stuff works! Not just because I have studied it and have seen the effects on my patients, but because it is what I use to look after myself. I can honestly say I feel great at the moment. But that hasn't always been the case. I have felt over-weight, stressed out, suffering with poor sleep, self-medicating every setback in life with excesses. A few years ago I had a horrible sense that life just wasn't fair and nothing was going to change. But then *I* changed. Not all at once, but slowly over time. I got involved with meditation and mindfulness first, which made the world of difference to how I felt on the inside. Mindfulness is about living in the moment and becoming more connected to how you feel in the present and your surroundings instead of constantly dwelling on the past or dreaming of the future. It also helped me to stop looking for outside forces to make me happy and I realised it all lies within me. This encouraged me to stop unhealthy 'fad diets' and focus on healthier lifestyle changes by increasing my fruit and vegetable intake, juicing and cutting down on sugar, which I do love! I now try and have my treats in moderation. I decided to party less, as I was just exhausted all the time and run-down. I used to feel I had to go out to prove how fun and funky I am, but I know now I don't have to prove anything to anyone and can just spend time doing things I enjoy.

I have stopped spending time with people who used me and sapped my energy and now prefer to have a few stronger supportive friendships. I can't always exercise as I often work up to 15 hours a day, but I try to go for walks at lunchtime and do my stretches in between patients. I am in a good place now, but it hasn't happened overnight. I made lots of little changes over a period of time to avoid being overwhelmed by it all and giving up, and I can honestly say it has made the world of difference. I know that the same can happen for you. My own experiences have led me to practise medicine in the way I do: by seeing an individual as a 'whole' and looking at all aspects of their life to gain optimum health. Of course I slip up from time to time because I get busy or eat too much chocolate for a few weeks and dodge going to the gym, but I realise that I am a work in progress and take time out to look after myself and try not to be too hard on myself. I remember why it is important to look after my health and simply start again.

Everything I recommend you try, I have already tried and tested on myself. I wouldn't expect you to do anything I wouldn't do. Trust me. Work with me and allow me to support you every step of the way. If there has been scientific research on recommendations mentioned in the book I will let you know. Together, we can achieve the very best energy, health and shape you could wish for. Let's get started!

CHAPTER 1
BECOME EMPOWERED

The state of health in the developed world is in crisis. People are living longer but in poorer health. Obesity, diabetes, strokes and heart attacks have reached epidemic proportions. Health services are struggling to cope and are, in some areas, at breaking point.

A study published in March 2013 showed that while we may all live until we are 80, we will be in poorer health and spending more time in ill health or in hospital.[1] This doesn't sound like much fun to me. As a GP, I go to lots of nursing homes and see elderly people who are bedbound or chronically ill, and having little pleasure or enjoyment in life. That's not the future I want.

While the NHS does a great job for a lot of people in the UK, many have become dependent on it and have forgotten that ultimately *we* are responsible for our own health. As a GP I find my patients fall into two categories in general. Some feel that if a treatment isn't available on the NHS it probably isn't any good and isn't worth paying for, and then there are those who believe in 'non-traditional' therapies, such as acupuncture and osteopathy, and are frustrated that the NHS doesn't cover more of them. In the UK, alternative therapies are often viewed with suspicion and derision, while the Americans and Australians offer them as a matter of course. People need to realise that our health service is doing a great job to treat immediate and serious health problems, such as heart attacks and strokes and diseases that require medications or surgery, but that we also have to make some provisions for our own well-being by making lifestyle changes and sometimes self-funding treatments to promote our own well-being and lower the chances of us getting ill in the first place. In order for the health service to run effectively, we all have to work to reduce the strain on it by taking responsibility for our own health and looking after ourselves as well as possible, so the sickest people are able to get the treatment they need in a timely fashion. I believe that even if you are born with a chronic health condition, you still have the power to improve your situation by making the right choices. In my opinion, there is simply no excuse.

Let me give you some examples of how integrative medicine can make a difference to health conditions. One of the pioneers of integrative health in the USA is Dr Dean Ornish. He devised a programme that is available throughout the US on health insurance plans which has been proven to reverse heart disease and prostate cancer. After following this plan, scans of the arteries have shown that the 'furring' that causes angina and heart attacks is reduced and reversed. Scans of patients' prostate glands show the cancer disappearing after they have followed this plan for several months. Would you like to know what this amazing plan is that can reverse heart disease and prostate cancer? It involves following a very low-fat vegetarian diet, doing yoga, meditation and being part of a support group. That's it. No invasive surgeries or harsh chemotherapy drugs.[2]

Here in the UK, another example is a gentleman called Allan Taylor. A 76-year-old grandfather, Mr Taylor was diagnosed with bowel cancer and had to undergo surgery and chemotherapy. He then went for his follow-up appointment and discovered the cancer had sadly reoccurred in a different part of the bowel. His doctors told him it was futile to have any more treatment as the cancer would keep reoccurring elsewhere and he was to only receive palliative care. Mr Taylor didn't settle for this grim prognosis. Following his own research on the Internet, he put himself on a programme that consisted of a vegetarian diet and having at least ten portions of fruit and vegetables a day, taking apricot kernels, selenium, powdered barley grass, turmeric capsules and high doses of vitamin C. Four months later Mr Taylor went for a scan and there was no trace of cancer in his body.[3]

Clearly the body can do wonderful things; we just need to give it the right fuel to do them.

IT'S IN MY GENES...

There is not a week that goes by that I don't hear this from a patient. But guess what? Amazing Nobel prize-winning research from 2009 showed that genes are not fixed as we once thought. The telomeres on the end of genes can be shortened or length-ened: the shorter your telomere, the more likely you are to age and shorten your lifespan; whereas the longer your telomere is, the longer your lifespan is. A lot of things that shorten your telo-meres are self-explanatory, like smoking, drinking too much or having a poor diet. The most surprising finding for me was that stress shortens your telomeres *as much as smoking does*. Therefore, stress is as bad for your health as smoking.[4]

Dr Dean Ornish found that within three months of patients taking part in his health programmes, there were changes in over five hundred genes – 'turning on' disease-preventing genes and 'turning off' disease-promoting genes that are involved in chronic diseases and cancers. Dr Ornish says that genes are a pre-disposition, but not your fate.

We often think of medical advances as new drugs, procedures and technology, but the truth is that simple choices like what we eat, how we manage our stress, how much exercise we get and how happy we feel makes a huge difference to our health and well-being.

OUR OWN INTERNAL SOURCE OF ENERGY

Every cell of our body is made of pure energy. When we are physically, emotionally and spiritually well the energy flows evenly through our bodies and we feel well and full of vitality. Many traditions such as yoga, Buddhism and Taoism work to restore the balance and flow of energy in our bodies. Chinese medicine and acupuncture work to restore our energy flow. The energies that run through our body are sometimes known as Chi, Auras, Chakras or Meridians. Chi is thought to be our pure source of energy that flows through us and gives us energy from within. Our Aura is the energy that surrounds us; Chakras are the energy centres that are found in the body and correspond to different organs and emotions. Meridians are the energy streams that flow through the body. When our energy is out of balance, it can affect our hormonal system, affect our circulation, disrupt the chemical signals in the body and affect our nervous system. The methods and techniques you learn in this book, be it what you eat, how you move your body or how you de-stress, will work to help you restore your internal sources of energy. Every cell in our body vibrates at a certain frequency and by eating well and doing other good things for our health we can replenish our own internal source of energy.

THE ENERGY HEALTH CHECK

To help you in your quest to improve your energy, this questionnaire assesses the different areas of your health that could be being affected. It has been designed in conjunction with Dr Mark Atkinson, an integrative medical physician and mindfulness teacher.[5] This will guide you to the chapters you need the most. Alternatively you could read the chapters and see which ones resound with you. Fill out the questionnaire and see which areas you score most highly in – this will help guide you in your personalised health plan.

1. FLUCTUATING BLOOD SUGAR LEVELS

In the last month have you: no = 0, occasionally = 1, yes = 2

1. Craved sweet foods or stimulants such as caffeine or nicotine? ____
2. Felt memory problems or mental confusion after eating? ____
3. Felt a drop in energy, mood or drowsiness after meals? ____
4. Experienced frequent mood swings in the course of a day? ____
5. Struggled with your weight despite watching what you eat? ____
6. Stored most of your body fat around your middle? ____
7. Felt weak? ____
8. Had a tendency to night sweats or excessive sweating during the day? ____
9. Experienced excessive thirst? ____

TOTAL SCORE: ____

2. ADRENAL FATIGUE

In the last month have you: no = 0, occasionally = 1, yes = 2

1. Felt stressed, restless, overwhelmed and/or exhausted? ____
2. Experienced anxiety, nervousness, irritability, phobias or panic attacks? ____
3. Kept yourself going on sugar, caffeine and/or snacks? ____
4. Experienced light-headedness on standing? ____
5. Felt more awake at night? ____
6. Craved salty food, sugar or liquorice? ____
7. Had dark circles under your eyes or feel your eyes sensitive to bright lights? ____
8. Spent the whole day rushing from one thing to another? ____
9. Suffered from interrupted sleep or insomnia? ____
10. Got absent-minded or felt that your short-term memory lets you down? ____

TOTAL SCORE: ____

3. OESTROGEN/PROGESTERONE IMBALANCE (WOMEN)

Do you: no = 0, occasionally = 1, yes = 2

1. Experience premenstrual mood swings? ___
2. Use, or have you used, birth control pills or hormone medication? ___
3. Experience irregular, lengthy or uncomfortable periods? ___
4. Experience peri- or post-menopausal discomfort (such as hot flushes, weight gain, sweats or insomnia)? ___
5. Have acne, excessive facial hair and/or are known to have Polycystic Ovary Syndrome (PCOS)? ___
6. Have a history of miscarriage or infertility? ___
7. Have painful or lumpy breasts? ___
8. Experience cyclical headaches or migraines? ___
9. Gain weight easily or find it hard to lose weight? ___

TOTAL SCORE: ___

4. LOW TESTOSTERONE QUESTIONNAIRE (MEN)

Do you: no = 0, occasionally = 1, yes = 2

1. Have any memory lapses, foggy thinking or periods of forgetfulness? ___
2. Have a reduced sex drive? ___
3. Experience problems with getting a firm erection? ___
4. Find that you are losing muscle mass and/or getting increased amounts of abdominal fat? ___
5. Experience apathy and low energy levels? ___
6. Find that you are experiencing increasing fatigue and deteriorating stamina? ___
7. Have enlargement of your breasts? ___
8. Experience any prostate problems, such as difficulty urinating, or poor urine stream? ___
9. Have depression? ___
10. Have joint stiffness, aches or pains that aren't related to arthritis? ___

TOTAL SCORE: ___

5. DYSBIOSIS - AN IMBALANCE OF BACTERIA IN THE GUT

In the last month have you: no = 0, occasionally = 1, yes = 2

1. Craved alcohol, sugar and/or bread?   ____
2. Experienced recurring digestive problems such as abdominal bloating, excessive wind, heartburn, diarrhoea or constipation?   ____
3. Got yeast infections, such as thrush?   ____
4. In the past have you had a diagnosis of yeast, candida and/or parasites?   ____
5. Experienced foggy headedness or unexplained migraines?   ____
6. Experienced unexplained tiredness, poor concentration and/or depression?   ____
7. Have you used steroids or birth control pills for more than one year?   ____
8. Had chronic fungus on your nails, skin or athlete's foot? ____
9. Had stools of an unusual colour, shape or consistency?   ____
10. Had any food allergies or intolerances?   ____

TOTAL SCORE: ____

6. TOXICITY

Do you: no = 0, occasionally = 1, yes = 2

1. Have any mercury amalgam fillings in your mouth?   ____
2. Have a weakened immune system or history of candida/parasites?   ____
3. Have a diagnosis of multiple sclerosis or an unexplained neurological disease?   ____
4. Have muscle weakness?   ____
5. Have unexplained neurological or mental health problems?   ____
6. Have short-term memory loss or Alzheimer's disease?   ____
7. Have a metallic taste in your mouth?   ____
8. Have dark spots on your gums or a swollen tongue?   ____

9. Eat canned food more than once a week? ___

TOTAL SCORE: ___

7. BODY ACIDIFICATION

Do you: no = 0, occasionally = 1, yes = 2
1. Have any chronic health problems? ___
2. Eat convenience, microwave and/or fast foods more than three times a week? ___
3. Rarely eat a minimum of five fruit and vegetables a day? ___
4. Have a tendency to be angry, get frustrated or hold resentment? ___
5. Have any problems with your liver or intestines? ___
6. Experience low energy levels? ___
7. Rarely exercise or make time to relax deeply? ___
8. Experience moderate to high levels of stress? ___
9. * Find it hard to recover from infections, or suspect your immune system is under-functioning? ___

TOTAL SCORE: ___

8. DIGESTIVE HEALTH IMBALANCE

Do you: no = 0, occasionally = 1, yes = 2
1. Have irritable bowel syndrome or inflammatory bowel disease? ___
2. Get intermittent or continuous diarrhoea or constipation? ___
3. Have a yeast infection such as thrush? ___
4. Experience foggy-headedness? ___
5. Have abdominal bloating, burping, indigestion or abdominal distension? ___
6. Experience tiredness or chronic fatigue? ___
7. Suspect that you might have problems absorbing nutrients? ___
8. Have any allergies or food intolerances? ___

TOTAL SCORE: ___

9. CHRONIC INFLAMMATION

Do you: no = 0, occasionally = 1, yes = 2

1. Have any inflammatory health conditions?
   (e.g., bowel problems/arthritis/infections)   ____
2. Have presently or previously a history of diabetes,
   cancer, heart disease or lupus?   ____
3. Have a waist size greater than 86cm (34 inches) for
   women or 102cm (40 inches) for men?   ____
4. Eat convenience, microwave and/or fast foods more
   than three times a week?   ____
5. Have bleeding gums?   ____
6. Have diabetes or syndrome X?   ____
7. Experience morning stiffness?   ____
8. Exercise vigorously and regularly?   ____
9. Experience moderate to high levels of stress?   ____

TOTAL SCORE: ____

10. PSYCHOLOGICAL STRESS

Do you: no = 0, occasionally = 1, yes = 2

1. Feel stressed out most of the time?   ____
2. Find it hard to cope with stressful situations?   ____
3. Live a stressful life?   ____
4. Find it hard not to worry about things?   ____
5. Struggle to manage your stress?   ____
6. Find it difficult to relax and enjoy your life?   ____
7. Think/know that stress is negatively affecting your
   health/life?   ____
8. Manage stress through the use of food, drink, smoking,
   gambling, drugs or sex?   ____
9. Get easily irritated, depressed, upset and/or anxious? ____

TOTAL SCORE: ____

RESULTS

The following guides you to which chapters to look at first if you score highly in the categories above:

1. Fluctuating blood sugar levels: chapters 4, 5, 6, 7, 8 and 10
2. Adrenal fatigue: chapters 4 and 11
3. Oestrogen progesterone imbalance (women): chapter 14
4. Low testosterone questionnaire (men): chapter 14
5. Dysbiosis: chapters 5 and 6
6. Toxicity: chapters 5, 7, 10 and 12
7. Body acidification: chapter 8
8. Digestive health imbalance: chapter 5
9. Chronic inflammation: chapters 3, 4, 5 and 12
10. Psychological stress: chapters 11 and 13

Now that you have worked out what is making you tired, it's time to get started and learn what you can do to achieve a healthier, happier and fatigue-free existence!

CHAPTER 2
MEDICAL CAUSES OF TIREDNESS

As a general practitioner, I see so many patients complaining about tiredness. I always examine them and arrange appropriate blood tests, but in the majority of cases I already know the results will come back completely normal. Sometimes, however, there *can* be a medical cause for tiredness. This chapter covers the most common causes. Savvy readers may wonder where the information about thyroid disorders is, but the thyroid gland and its disorders are such a big topic that they have their own separate chapter (see page 33). If you're concerned about any of the conditions outlined below then please see your doctor for further advice and investigations.

IRON-DEFICIENCY ANAEMIA

One of the most common reasons for feeling tired and run-down is iron-deficiency anaemia. It affects around one in 20 men and post-menopausal women, but it is even more common in women who have periods. Women with heavy periods or who are pregnant often become anaemic. Iron-deficiency anaemia can also be caused by a stomach ulcer or by taking too many non-steroidal anti-inflammatory drugs (NSAIDS), such as aspirin or ibuprofen, which can damage the lining of the stomach and intestines.[1]

The typical symptoms are feeling tired, lethargic and unmotivated, having aching muscles and getting worn out easily after doing everyday activities such as your job and household chores. A blood test can confirm iron-deficiency anaemia, by checking your full blood count (FBC) and ferritin level. Ferritin is the protein form in which iron is stored in the body.

If a blood test confirms a diagnosis of iron-deficiency anaemia, iron supplements can help boost the blood count, alongside a diet consisting of iron-rich foods such as dark-green leafy vegetables, curly kale and spinach, beans, nuts, dark meat and dried fruit. For some people, iron supplements prescribed by doctors can cause constipation or stomach discomfort, and almost always turn your stools very dark or black. If this is not tolerable for you, health-food stores often sell milder alternatives that boost your iron in a slower way but with less side effects. Drinking more than two or three strong cups of tea and coffee per day makes it harder

The holistic approach

A normal level of ferritin covers a wide range and can vary from laboratory to laboratory so it is best to check with your doctor what it is when looking at your own results, but it is usually from approximately 12 to 150 mg/mL. It does vary between men and women too. If I see a patient who's feeling very tired and has a level below 90, I advise that they take a food-based iron supplement such as spirulina or increase foods in their diet that are rich in iron. Even though they may fall into the normal range, meaning they have a sufficient iron level to function, their level is still at the lower end and I prefer my patients' bodies to be functioning optimally, not just sufficiently.

to absorb iron due to the tannins in these drinks, as does a lot of calcium in the diet, for example if you consume a lot of dairy products like milk, and medications like antacids for heartburn and indigestion.

If you develop iron-deficiency anaemia for the first time and are aged over 55, your doctor will probably want to arrange some more tests to make sure this is not a sign of an underlying illness or condition.

ANAEMIA DUE TO A FOLATE OR VITAMIN B12 DEFICIENCY

A deficiency of vitamin B12 or folate can cause the red blood cells to become abnormally large and unable to function properly, leading to symptoms of tiredness and lethargy. Vitamin B12 and folate work together to make healthy red blood cells. In addition, vitamin B12 keeps the neurological system – brain, nerves and spinal cord – healthy, and folate is very important for pregnant women to prevent birth and spinal cord defects in the unborn foetus. This type of anaemia is diagnosed with a blood test, checking the FBC, vitamin B12 and folate levels.[2]

Treating these anaemias is fairly straightforward. Folic acid supplements are taken to restore folate levels, which usually takes three to four months. If there is a vitamin B12 deficiency, you can normally have a course of injections first to restore the balance, and then either a course of supplements or further injections every few months. Improving your diet can also help. Natural food sources of vitamin B12 are eggs, meat and dairy products, and folate food sources are green vegetables such as broccoli, Brussels sprouts and peas. Spirulina supplements are also rich in vitamin B12.

Vitamin B12 and folate deficiencies are more common in the over-75s, affecting approximately one in 10 people. In younger people it can be due to a diet lacking in fruit and vegetables.

Pernicious anaemia is a type of vitamin B12 anaemia that affects approximately one in 10,000 people in Northern Europe. It's caused by a lack of absorption of vitamin B12 in the intestines due to a lack of a secretion called intrinsic factor, thought to be an autoimmune disease.[3]

DIABETES MELLITUS

Diabetes is a long-term and serious condition caused by too much sugar in the blood. If left untreated or uncontrolled it can cause serious complications such as kidney problems, blindness and even the loss of a limb. One of the first symptoms can be feeling tired. The other key symptoms are feeling very thirsty, going to the toilet to pass urine a lot more than usual and unexplained weight loss. Your doctor can diagnose diabetes with a blood test so do visit your doctor if you are concerned.

Some people are born with diabetes as their body does not produce enough insulin to process sugars, and this is known as type 1 diabetes mellitus. Most people who develop diabetes in later life do so because the pancreas, which produces insulin, becomes 'worn out' and can no longer produce enough insulin to deal with the levels of sugars in the body. The pancreas generally becomes worn out due to overuse, that is, there has been too much sugar consumed over time and it can no longer produce enough insulin to cope with the amounts of sugar being ingested. This is commonly known as type 2 diabetes mellitus.

Many people with type 2 diabetes mellitus do produce some insulin, just not enough to cope with the levels of sugar in the body. There are medications that can be prescribed to help boost the function of the cells in the pancreas to produce more insulin, but another way to deal with this is to modify your diet.

The holistic approach

I have seen many patients with diabetes able to control it without medication by following a very strict diet. This involves cutting out almost all the sugar in your diet and reducing all processed foods and in general, 'eating clean'. Sugar is added to most processed foods, as well as bread and milk, which is why people with diabetes need to strictly control the amounts of these foods that they eat. You will find out more about this in chapter 6 and more information about eating clean in chapters 8 and 9. It is also important to lose weight and cut out bad habits like smoking, as having diabetes increases your risk of heart attacks and strokes. It is entirely possible to control diabetes without medications and reduce the chances of long-term complications as long as you are willing to make changes for the benefit of your health.

SLEEP APNOEA

Sleep apnoea is a condition where the muscles in the neck fail to keep the airways open causing the throat to narrow during sleep and repeatedly interrupt breathing. This subsequently causes a drop in the blood's oxygen levels and the constant interrupted sleep can therefore make you feel tired.

Symptoms of sleep apnoea include snoring, waking up with a headache, feeling moody, nasal congestion and extreme tiredness in the day. A lot of people don't realise they suffer from this and have no idea why they are waking up so often in the night. It is normally brought to the person's attention when they share a bedroom with someone else. If someone has ever told you that you stop breathing in your sleep for brief periods, this is probably the reason why. The major cause for this is being overweight, and so losing weight has to be the priority for people with this condition and is the best holistic advice I can offer for this condition. Other more invasive treatments are available such as sleep masks and other devices that work to keep your airways open, and your doctor can give you more detailed information.

COELIAC DISEASE

This is a type of food intolerance where the body fails to digest gluten, a substance found in cakes, bread, cereal and pasta, to name a few. There are 250,000 cases in the UK, but researchers believe that up to 90 per cent of sufferers are unaware they have an intolerance. Symptoms include tiredness, diarrhoea, bloating, abdominal pains, anaemia and weight loss. It can be diagnosed by your doctor by a blood test, to measure the anti-tissue trans-glutaminase antibodies (anti-tTG). If these are high it indicates coeliac disease.[4] The treatment involves a very strict gluten-free diet to keep symptoms at bay and stop the disease from worsening. Gluten is found in grains such as wheat, barley and rye, meaning foods such as bread, cereals, cakes, cookies, pasta, beer, most ready-made sauces, soups and salad dressings and chips are out.

In my experience, many patients have the symptoms of coeliac disease but negative blood tests. In these cases, they may have a gluten sensitivity rather than coeliac disease and so I advise them to have a period of total abstinence from gluten-rich foods and then limit them to only once or twice a week. This is because gluten-sensitive individuals can only cope with small amounts of gluten and not the daily bombardment that is common to most of us.

GLANDULAR FEVER

This is a common viral infection that causes fatigue, fever, sore throat and swollen glands. It's common in teenagers and young adults but can happen in later years too. The sore throat and swollen gland symptoms usually resolve in weeks, but the lethargy can continue for months. Once again, this can be discovered with a blood test, looking for antibodies. There is no specific treatment for this condition other than rest and rehydration. It can be helpful to support the body to heal as much as possible by consuming plenty of fruit and vegetables for the nutrient value, adding a good-quality multivitamin and taking extra vitamin C and zinc to help boost the immune system.

DEPRESSION AND ANXIETY

As well as feeling low in mood, it is common to feel drained of energy and lethargic when depressed. One of the symptoms of depression is difficulty sleeping and waking up in the early hours, which inevitably causes more tiredness during the day.

People who suffer from anxiety can often feel worried, irritable and tired.

If your mood is affecting your energy levels it would be worthwhile seeking medical help. There are lots of options to help treat anxiety and depression, ranging from medication to counselling to herbal treatments and natural remedies. The key is to find a treatment that works well for you and fits in with your ethos and lifestyle. Exercise has been proven to improve mood as much as antidepressant medication in some cases, and it is also important to eat healthily as fluctuating blood sugars can make depression and anxiety worse and the body needs B vitamins and fish oils to balance your mood.

FIBROMYALGIA

Fibromyalgia is a condition that causes widespread pain and extreme tiredness. Ninety per cent of sufferers are women. It's estimated that there are one in 20 sufferers worldwide, and approximately 1.76 million adults affected in the United Kingdom. Fibromyalgia can develop at any age, but it's most common to appear between the ages of 30–60. Other symptoms include headaches, irritable bowel syndrome, poor sleep patterns and muscle stiffness. People with this condition often get 'fibro-fog', which can affect speech, cause attention and concentration problems, and cause difficulty with memory and learning new things. Other symptoms can be depression, feeling too hot or too cold, tingling or numbness or burning in the hands and feet and painful menstrual cycles in women.

Unfortunately no one knows what causes fibromyalgia but it's believed to be due to disrupted pain signalling in the body, hormone disruptions and sleep problems. Sometimes a period of emotional stress or trauma can precipitate the symptoms. It's quite a hard condition to diagnose as the symptoms are not very specific. It often becomes a diagnosis of exclusion, meaning tests are carried out to rule out other medical conditions and ensure there is no alternative diagnosis.

The criteria for diagnosing fibromyalgia are:

- widespread pain for more than three months in all four quadrants of the body, that is on both the right and left sides of the body, above and below the waist.
- pain in at least 11 of the 18 'tender points' when they are pressed. These tender points are classically on the neck, on the top of the back, between the neck and the chest, above each of the shoulder blades, inside the elbows, above and below the buttocks on both sides and the knees.

Once fibromyalgia is diagnosed, there is no specific treatment other than symptom control. This means that the pain can be managed with medication, treating any depression that may be associated with the condition and some physical therapy to help relieve the muscle pains.[5]

The holistic approach

I would not diagnose a patient of mine with fibromyalgia until they had made major lifestyle changes first. This would include yoga and stretching, relaxation exercises like deep breathing and mindfulness, and trying the three-week cleanse plan (chapter 9), changing their diet and cutting out alcohol and smoking. With my own clients, the majority of their symptoms resolve within three months. In fact, my dad and I once went through the diagnostic criteria for fibromyalgia and we both had it! This was because I had had several weeks of excess and partying and was run-down and had done no exercise and had a poor diet, and my dad is getting a bit older and more achy. (Sorry, Dad!)

Matt is a 36-year-old man who had been diagnosed with fibromyalgia after having several months of aches and pains, lethargy and stress. His doctor told him he would never work again. He came to see me as he was under-standably not happy with this diagnosis. Matt didn't look after his health at all, and had forgotten that there's a major connection between what we ingest and how we feel. He also had a lot of work and personal stress. After just one month of working with me to create a health plan which included an intensive change in his eating patterns, cutting down on sugar, smoking and alcohol, gentle stretching, looking at ways of managing his stress and dealing with issues in his life that were causing him conflict, he felt 90 per cent better and was able to go back to work full time. That was over a year ago and Matt is still well and happy and has gone on to get a new better job and start a family. In my experience, lifestyle changes are often enough to resolve these symptoms in the majority of cases.

CHRONIC FATIGUE SYNDROME

Chronic fatigue syndrome (CFS) is also known as ME or myalgic encephalomyelitis. Myalgia means muscle pain and encephalomyelitis means inflammation of the brain and spinal cord. This term is not used so commonly by health-care professionals nowadays as there's no evidence of any inflammation of the brain and spinal cord with this condition.

It is estimated that 250,000 people in the UK have CFS.[6] It is more common in women than in men and usually develops in the early 20s to mid-40s. Like fibromyalgia, the exact cause is unknown. Proposed causes are a viral infection, a problem with the immune system, a hormonal imbalance, or stress and emotional trauma. There is also some thought that genetics could make a person more susceptible.

The symptoms are variable and widespread, but the main symptom is a persistent fatigue that affects the sufferer both physically and mentally. Exercise can make the fatigue worse, and it may come on several hours or the next day after doing exercise. People with severe CFS struggle to do normal everyday activities such as wash and dress themselves. Other symptoms can include muscle and joint pains, headaches, poor short-term memory and concentration, stomach pains like irritable bowel syndrome (IBS), sore throat, poor sleep, psychological difficulties like depression, irritability and panic attacks, painful lymph nodes and sensitivity or intolerance to light, loud noises, alcohol and certain foods. Less common symptoms are dizziness, excessive sweating, difficulty controlling body temperature and balance problems.

CFS takes a long time to be diagnosed as other conditions with similar symptoms first need to be ruled out. Examples of this are having blood tests to rule out anaemia, thyroid dysfunction, liver or kidney problems. Depression can sometimes mimic the symptoms of CFS too.

The National Institute for Health and Care Excellence (NICE) issued guidance in 2007 that stated that doctors should consider diagnosing CFS if a person has fatigue and all of the following:

- it is new or had a clear starting point. That is, it has not been a lifelong problem
- it is persistent and/or recurrent
- it is unexplained by other conditions
- it substantially reduces the amount of activity someone can do
- it feels worse after physical activity

The person should also have one or more of these symptoms:

- difficulty sleeping, or insomnia
- muscle or joint pain without inflammation
- headaches
- painful lymph nodes that are not enlarged
- sore throat
- poor mental function, such as difficulty thinking
- symptoms getting worse after physical or mental exertion
- feeling unwell or having flu-like symptoms
- dizziness or nausea
- heart palpitations without heart disease

CFS can be diagnosed after other conditions have been ruled out and the above symptoms have persisted for at least four months in an adult and three months in a child.

There is no cure for CFS, treatment is targeted at relieving symptoms.

MANAGING CHRONIC FATIGUE SYNDROME

Below are some of the common recommendations made to patients about managing their CFS:

Cognitive Behavioural Therapy (CBT) aims to reduce the severity of the symptoms and the distress associated with CFS by breaking down problems into smaller parts and by breaking the negative cycle around thoughts, feelings, physical sensations and actions.

Graded exercise therapy is a structured exercise programme that aims to gradually increase how long a person can carry out a physical activity. It usually involves exercises such as walking or swimming. There are specialist therapists who are experienced in doing graded exercise with people with CFS. They work with the individual to find their baseline level for exercise and then work to gradually increase the time doing the exercise and the intensity. The aim of the exercise programme is to set goals such as being able to walk to the shops or do housework for 20 minutes. It may take a long time to achieve the goals, but it is important to follow the graded exercise plan.

Activity management involves setting individual goals and gradually increasing the activity levels in a way that the person finds manageable. A therapist may suggest keeping a diary of the individual's current activities and rest periods to establish what their baseline is. Activities will then be increased gradually in a way that the person can manage.

Medication can be used to relieve the symptoms of CFS. Painkillers can be used to ease muscle and joint pains or headaches. If a person suffers with long-term pain, their doctor can refer them to a pain management clinic for further intervention, which usually involves medication, alternative therapies for pain management such as acupuncture, psychological support and relaxation techniques. Antidepressants can be useful for people with CFS who are feeling depressed, or are in pain and have trouble sleeping. A commonly used drug is called amitriptyline, a low-grade tricyclic antidepressant, but the side effects can be intolerable to some people as they can include dry mouth, blurred vision, dizziness and drowsiness. Anti-sickness medication can help those who suffer from nausea. There is no specific medication that can treat CFS.

Other recommended self-help techniques are avoiding stress, eating small regular meals to avoid nausea, relaxation and trying not to sleep excessively or napping as this does not improve the sleep problems.

The holistic approach

As with fibromyalgia, I would not make this diagnosis until my client had made drastic lifestyle changes. These would include a change in diet, avoiding alcohol, smoking, sugar, sweeteners, taking up gentle exercise such as yoga and stretching, managing stress with breathing exercises, mindfulness and other relaxation techniques. I have found that high dose supplementation of vitamins and minerals, sometimes given intravenously, can boost a person's immune system and improve their symptoms.

I definitely believe the symptoms the individual experiences are real and disabling, but unlike conventional medicine, I know that in the majority of cases there is an underlying imbalance – be it emotional, physical, chemical, vitamin and mineral or hormonal. Unlike conventional medicine, which just makes the diagnosis and then manages symptoms, my integrative approach means that I work with my clients to find imbalances and treat them, resolving the symptoms so my clients can get back to their normal lives, functioning well. A really good start would be to do the three-week energy cleanse outlined in chapter 9 as in the majority of cases this will improve symptoms. This approach involves a lot of hard work from the individual and I admit it can be very difficult, even causing temporary psychological distress, but if they want to get better, their total engagement and commitment is needed to facilitate the process. And, of course, it's worth it to live a full and healthy life.

CHAPTER 3
THYROID DISORDERS

The thyroid is a small, butterfly-shaped gland that sits at the front of the neck and is really important for energy regulation. It produces thyroid hormones which are secreted into the bloodstream and then act as messengers, affecting cells and tissues and regulating many processes in the body. We can use the analogy of a car when talking about the thyroid hormones: when the thyroid gland is working properly, the car is driving smoothly and there's just the right amount of pressure on the accelerator pedal. Within the body the thyroid hormones regulate our metabolism, keep our energy levels high, aid good sleep, regulate our bowels and aid digestion.

When the thyroid hormones are not balanced and are running too high, it's akin to pushing down hard on the accelerator. This leads to symptoms such as diarrhoea, agitation, light or no periods, hunger, disrupted sleep, fast speech and a 'hyper' mood. When the thyroid gland is sluggish and underactive, it's similar to pushing down on the brakes of the car. The individual will feel sleepy, tired, low in mood, have long heavy periods, be constipated, gain weight and have a low appetite. They can also have dry skin and their hair can become thin or fall out.

In this chapter I'm going to talk about when the thyroid gland is underactive as one of the main symptoms of this is tiredness, otherwise known as hypothyroidism. I will also talk about how to manage when the thyroid is functioning less than optimally, and what actions and medications can help. When your thyroid gland is over-functioning, known as hyperthyroidism, tiredness is not a problem, in fact, the sufferers almost have too much energy and feel jittery and cannot sleep. There are also other associated health problems with the condition.

HOW TO DIAGNOSE HYPOTHYROIDISM

Hypothyroidism should be diagnosed by a combination of blood tests and the observation of clinical symptoms the patient is experiencing. As outlined above, common symptoms are tiredness, weak hair and nails, dry skin, constipation, lack of periods, low appetite and weight gain.

The thyroid gland makes two hormones called thyroxine (T4) and triiodothyronine (T3). In order to make T3 and T4, the body needs a good amount of iodine. In the body most of T4 is inactive and is converted into T3, which is the most active thyroid hormone.

The activity of the thyroid gland and the production of both T3 and T4 are controlled by hormones produced in two parts of the brain called the hypothalamus and the pituitary. The hypothalamus detects information about the various states of bodily functions. When the hypothalamus detects that levels of T3 and T4 are low, it releases a hormone called thyrotropin-releasing hormone (TRH). TRH then travels to the pituitary gland and stimulates it to release a hormone called thyroid-stimulating hormone (TSH). TSH then moves into the bloodstream and travels to the thyroid gland causing cells in the gland to make more T3 and T4 and release it into the bloodstream. This increases the metabolic rate of the cells as well as carrying out other roles in the body. When there are sufficiently high levels of T3 and T4 in the body, this is detected by the pituitary gland and hypothalamus and the production of TSH and TRH is stopped. This type of feedback mechanism ensures the body always has optimum levels of the thyroid hormones and is illustrated below:

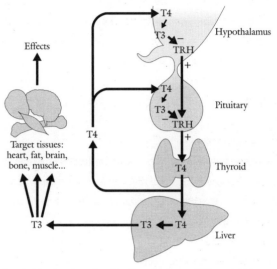

Feedback Mechanism for the Production of Thyroid Hormones
– The Hypothalmic-Pituitary-Thyroid Axis

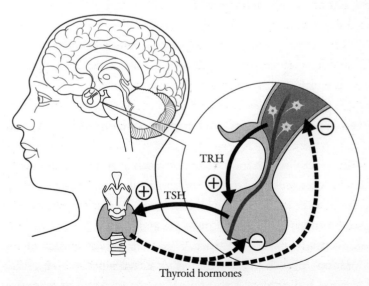

Thyroid hormones

Feedback Mechanism for the Production of Thyroid Hormones
– The Hypothalmic-Pituitary-Thyroid Axis

A thyroid hormone blood test measures the TSH level and T4 level routinely. T3 should also be measured routinely as its effects are more potent than that of T4. T4 is also converted to T3, and if there's a problem with this conversion this can result in a normal T4 level but a low T3 level. As T4 is not as potent as T3, this could explain why your blood levels of T4 may be normal but you still feel tired and sluggish.

There are a group of thyroid antibodies that are not routinely measured but I measure them in my patients. The most frequent antibodies seen are:

- Antithyroid Peroxidase Antibody otherwise known as Antithyroid Microsomal Antibody, or TPO Ab for short
- Antithyroglobulin Antibody or TG Ab
- Thyroid Stimulating Immunoglobulin or TSI Ab

TSI Ab stimulates the thyroid gland to overproduce thyroid hormones. This is known as Graves' Disease which is an autoimmune form of hyperthyroidism.

Both TPO Ab and TG Ab decrease thyroid function. Sometimes people can have elevated levels of these antibodies but have no clinical symptoms. In these cases regular monitoring, at least every six months, should be carried out.

IODINE AND THYROID FUNCTION

Iodine is very important for the functioning of the thyroid gland. This is because both T3 and T4 hormones made by the thyroid gland are high in iodine content, so if this isn't present, the thyroid gland cannot make the hormones and this will subsequently lead to tiredness and low energy levels. If you are experiencing symptoms of poor thyroid function then you could be iodine deficient. Iodine deficiency is one of the three most common nutritional deficiencies, along with magnesium and vitamin D.

More than 100 years ago, iodine was shown to reverse and prevent the swelling of the thyroid gland, also known as a goitre, and correct hypothyroidism. Iodine has other effects such as improving fertility, helping brain development in children, stabilising metabolism and body weight and optimising immune function. It is a potent anti-bacterial, anti-parasitic, anti-viral and anti-cancer agent and protects other organs and tissues in the body. For example, studies have shown that rates of breast cancer and fibrocystic breast disease, which is not cancerous but common, decrease with iodine supplementation.[1, 2]

Iodine and iodine-rich foods have a history of being natural treatments of hypertension and cardiovascular disease.[3] Studies have also shown that people living in iodine-deficient areas have higher rates of stomach cancers and increased iodine intake has been associated with a reduction in stomach cancer rates.[4, 5]

Iodine can be substituted in forms of supplements or by eating foods rich in iodine. The food with the most iodine in it is seaweed such as kelp or spirulina. Iodine, but less of it than in seaweed, is found in cod, baked potatoes with the skin, salt, shrimp, turkey breasts, tuna and eggs. The body cannot store iodine which is why a daily regular intake is needed. A maximum daily dose of 1.1mg (1100mcg) iodine is currently recommended but a dose of 150mcg, if someone is not deficient, is the recommended daily dose.

Your holistic health-care practitioner would be able to test your iodine levels if this is something you are concerned about. Some people who have overactive autoimmune thyroid conditions like Graves' disease should avoid iodine supplementation and rarely some people react to iodine. It's important to remember that excessive intake of iodine can also cause thyroid problems.

MEDICATION AND
THE THYROID GLAND

The most common medication prescribed for hypothyroidism is called levothyroxine. It's a synthetic thyroid hormone, meaning it's made in a laboratory. This substitutes T4 in the body. However, as mentioned earlier, if there's a problem converting T4 to T3 then this might not fully resolve symptoms. There are other types of thyroid medication, but these are not always widely available and sometimes can only be acquired through private practitioners. An example of this is a synthetic type of T3 or a synthetic combination of T3 and T4, like novothyral.

Armour is a natural combination of T3 and T4. The term 'natural' means non-synthetic, as the hormones are extracted from animals. These animals are normally bred for food as well as extracting the hormone. There have been arguments over whether synthetic or natural hormones are best. Some endocrinologists (specialist doctors who deal with hormonal imbalances) prefer synthetic hormones as the dose can be better controlled and each pill has a consistent dose, but some patients say they feel the natural medication works better and helps them control their symptoms better.

If you have been diagnosed with hypothyroidism and are not feeling better it could be that you need a different type of medication to suit your body better.

SYMPTOMS OF HYPOTHYROIDISM
DESPITE NORMAL BLOOD TESTS

Many people with the symptoms of hypothyroidism have normal thyroid blood tests. This can be for a variety of reasons. In my experience it can often be due to a dietary deficiency. Another reason you may be experiencing symptoms of low thyroid function could be because the normal range of the thyroid hormones is so wide. When the hormones are tested, the normal range of T4 is 12–22 pmol/l. It could be that your thyroid function is 12, which technically means it's normal, but you might not be feeling as well as someone who has a T4 level of 20 or more. In these circumstances I try and encourage my patients to make lifestyle and dietary changes to improve their thyroid function for a minimum of four months before re-testing to see if there's an improvement. If someone is still having strong thyroid symptoms despite making drastic changes to their life-style and has a T4 level around 12–13, then I would consider treating with medication. If you are already on thyroid medication and still don't feel well, it could be a case of needing a different medication, for example a medication that is a combination of T3 and T4 or just T3.

It could be that you have another imbalance in the body. Reading the rest of this book and seeing how to make changes in other areas in your body, such as in your adrenal glands or female hormones, and following the cleanse programme will help. If symptoms persist or you have any concerns then go and see your doctor or holistic practitioner for further input.

Kay, 40, had ongoing symptoms of tiredness, weight gain, lethargy, dry skin, dry hair and brittle nails. We tested her thyroid function and her T4 was 12. This is technically normal. We tried lifestyle changes and nutritional changes, but her T4 remained at 12 and she did not feel any better. We started a very low dose of levothyroxine at 25mcg and she felt a lot better within two months. Her T4 level went up to 16 so we decided to continue with this dose long term with regular blood monitoring. Kay understands that based on blood tests she does not have hypo-thyroidism, but is happy to take the medication as she feels better for doing so.

NUTRITIONAL SUPPORT
FOR THE THYROID GLAND

As well as increasing iodine in your diet, or through supplements, there are other nutritional changes that can be made to support the optimum functioning of the thyroid gland, and therefore increasing your energy levels. Selenium is important for thyroid function as it helps T4 convert to T3. Sufficient amounts of selenium can be obtained from the diet by having one or two Brazil nuts a day or by eating garlic. Magnesium is also important for the proper absorption of iodine and can be found in leafy green vegetables and whole grains. B vitamins, specifically vitamins B2 and B3, are needed to help the body use iodine at a cellular level. Vitamin D is important for the immune system so is very important in Hashimoto's and Graves' disease. It would also be beneficial to optimise your levels of omega-3 fatty acids, tyrosine, vitamin A and zinc. I advise reducing gluten or wheat if you have intolerances. Doing a detox or cleanse programme such as the energy cleanse is going to optimise your body to peak nutritional condition, as well as exercising, managing stress and taking saunas to aid detoxification and supplements, if needed, to support your nutritional needs.

Kelly is a 28-year-old woman who I saw with symptoms of tiredness, low mood and weight gain. Her thyroid function tests revealed a T4 level of 14. I put her on the three-week cleanse programme and advised taking supplements. She also started exercising and managing her stress more effectively. After four months she felt a lot better in herself and had much improved energy levels. Her T4 level was retested and had gone up to 17. The lifestyle and nutritional changes she made improved her symptoms and showed up biochemically on her blood tests too.

ACTION PLAN

If you are concerned that your thyroid gland is not functioning well it could be worth getting your TSH, T4 and T3 levels checked. Remember, not all NHS GPs are able to do these tests so you may have to have them done privately. If you want to try to naturally boost the functioning of your thyroid gland you can look at your diet, making sure you get enough iodine, selenium, vitamin D, magnesium and B vitamins in your food or with supplements.

CHAPTER 4
ADRENAL FATIGUE

ARE YOU RUNNING ON EMPTY?

The most common reasons people consult a GP are exhaustion, poor energy, low mood and restless sleep. Patients often are examined and subsequent investigations come back normal, yet their symptoms persist and affect their daily lives. Adrenal fatigue is a major cause of tiredness and lack of energy, but is a condition unrecognised and not taught to most conventional medical doctors, despite being recognised by the World Health Organization in 2010. Let me tell you about one case that sums up how many people feel:

Thirty-year-old Jane was constantly exhausted. When the alarm went off each morning, she would despair and 'snooze' it three or four times. Subsequently she was often late for work, having to rush to get ready with no time for breakfast, leaving the house only with a giant flask of coffee. The bags under her eyes were getting bigger and her skin more sallow. She would power through her work, swigging coffee, and by mid-morning she was starving.

Seeing as she hadn't had any breakfast, she would 'treat' herself to a large baguette for lunch, with crisps and a chocolate bar. After a short-lived high, she would crash again and grab more coffee, or if really struggling, a fizzy drink. She'd feel like she was wading through treacle all afternoon at work, drive home on auto-pilot, counting the hours until she could go to sleep.

Back at home, Jane was too exhausted to go out or do anything productive. She would sit on the sofa watching mindless TV shows or get lost in Facebook. However, when bedtime came she was more alert than she'd been all day, and spent hours tossing and turning before falling asleep around 2 a.m. The whole cycle would start again the next day with the dreaded sound of the alarm clock.

When the weekend came Jane would then sleep most of Saturday to 'catch up', feel good for that one afternoon and have enough energy to go out and party that night. The vicious cycle would start again on Sunday when her overindulgence the night before would leave her feeling fatigued all day and then, after a lazy day, unable to sleep again.

This case perfectly sums up how adrenal fatigue feels and how it affects a person's life.

The adrenals are two small glands that sit on top of the kidneys, each about the size of a walnut. Despite being small, they are very important for health and well-being. The adrenals affect virtually every system in our body. They aid our bodies in responding to stress, maintaining energy, regulating the immune system and our heart rate. They also maintain levels of minerals and keep blood sugar, fluid levels and blood pressure within a healthy range. They produce adrenaline and noradrenaline: the so-called 'fight or flight' hormones which help the body deal with acute stress. These are the hormones that give a person super-human strength, such as to lift up a car when a child is trapped underneath or the energy to run away from an attacker. The adrenal glands manufacture over 30 different steroids including cortisol, DHEA and cortisone which help the body control fats, proteins, carbohydrates, regulate insulin levels, reduce inflamma-tion and influence the immune system.

When the adrenal glands are healthy, they secrete precise amounts of the steroid hormones. However, too much physical, emotional, environmental or psychological stress causes imbalances in their functioning. This can result in adrenal fatigue, when the adrenal glands are no longer coping with the strains put on them. The classic symptoms are tiredness, low energy, cravings, insomnia, irritability, anxiety and poor concentration. Many people with adrenal fatigue get into the habit of relying on stimulants like caffeine and sugar to keep them going as they feel so fatigued in the day, and then alcohol or other relaxants to wind down at the end of the day as they have trouble switching off at night.[1]

There can be many causes of adrenal fatigue, such as work pressures, emotional traumas, relationship strains, chronic illness, infections, surgery, pain, grief, financial difficulties, lack of sleep or depression and anxiety.

SYMPTOMS OF ADRENAL FATIGUE

Do you:

1. Feel tired for no obvious reason?
2. Experience light-headedness on standing?
3. Feel more awake at night?
4. Crave salty foods, sugar or liquorice?
5. Feel stressed, restless, overwhelmed or exhausted?
6. Find it hard to lose weight?
7. Get absentminded or feel that your short-term memory lets you down?
8. Keep yourself going on sugar, caffeine and/or nicotine?
9. Spend the whole day rushing from one thing to another?
10. Experience anxiety, irritability or nervousness?
11. Have a low libido?
12. Suffer from interrupted sleep or insomnia?

If you answered yes to many of these questions you might have adrenal fatigue.

If a patient was to see me and ask for the adrenal gland to be checked, there are tests available to measure the DHEA and cortisol in a saliva sample. These would be taken at four different times over a 24-hour period. The levels would then be measured and compared to healthy controls. There are many nutritionists, naturopaths and doctors with similar training to myself who would be able to carry these tests out for you. A reputable company that can carry out this testing is listed in the Resources on page 239.

If you have access to a blood pressure monitoring device, you could try this: lie down for five minutes, check your blood pressure and record the result. Keep the blood pressure cuff on, stand up and immediately record your blood pressure again. The top figure of the reading should normally increase or stay the same. If it drops, it could be an indicator of adrenal fatigue. Repeat the test twice to confirm results.

The steroid hormone DHEA, which contributes to energy levels, can also be measured as a blood test to see if levels are within normal range. If the levels of DHEA come back as low then you could be suffering from an adrenal imbalance.

Are your looks suffering?

As well as causing an increase in your belly fat and dark circles around the eyes, when you suffer from adrenal fatigue your skin suffers too. The body is wasting so much energy keeping the adrenals going that it's no longer able to deliver nutrients to your skin. Over time, having adrenal fatigue will accelerate the ageing process and have you looking old before your time, unless you take steps to heal it.

CONVENTIONAL MEDICINE AND ADRENAL FATIGUE

Conventional mainstream medicine doesn't recognise adrenal fatigue and doctors are not taught about it in medical school. Adrenal fatigue was discovered by Dr James Wilson, the co-founder of the Canadian College of Naturopathic Medicine, in 1998, who believed that two-thirds of the North American population were suffering from it. He noticed a lot of his patients had common symptoms of tiredness, trouble getting up in the morning, reliance on coffee, colas, salty or sweet snacks, feeling run-down and stressed out. He also called it '21st-Century Syndrome'.[2] There is no concrete scientific evidence in support of a diagnosis of adrenal fatigue, however, the salivary tests do indicate abnormal cortisol secretion when tested. I believe it is a real phenomenon, especially as I have suffered myself due to an erratic lifestyle. Other adrenal conditions of imbalance are recognised like Cushing's syndrome (too much cortisol) and Addison's disease (too little cortisol, aldosterone and/or sex hormones).

So, it's all very well knowing your adrenals aren't working well, but how do you fix them?

HOW TO HEAL ADRENAL FATIGUE

As I say throughout this book, lifestyle changes hold the key to improving your health, and adrenal fatigue is no different. The following steps are things you can do yourself and are not costly. A lot of these steps will be considered in more detail throughout the book.

1. IDENTIFY AND RESOLVE YOUR MAIN SOURCES OF STRESS

When stress is our predominant state, our bodies will try to protect us by storing fat. We need to reduce stress to coax our bodies away from 'crisis mode'.

Go through your main causes of stress and identify a solution, for example if you have a lot of debt you might plan to discuss this with your local Citizens Advice Bureau, or if you have problems at work you might organise a meeting with your boss. Make a list of actions and put timeframes on them. It's important to take practical steps to improve your situation. If you need professional help, making an appointment to see your doctor would be a great first step.

How stress can make you fat

When you are stressed, your body sends a message to the adrenal glands to release more cortisol. Cortisol stops the hormone leptin being produced. Leptin sends signals that make us feel full. Without it we are prone to over-eating, and this absence makes us crave foods rich in carbohydrates in particular. When we experience long-term stress, cortisol and insulin remain high in the blood, and the extra glucose that isn't needed for energy gets stored in the form of fat – primarily *abdominal* fat cells. Scientists have discovered that fat cells have special stress-hormone receptors for cortisol, but there also seem to be more of these cortisol receptors on the fat cells around the stomach than anywhere else in the body.

---

2. EAT YOUR WAY BACK TO ENERGY

Eating regular meals throughout the day will stop your blood sugars and hormones from fluctuating too much. When we have a big meal cortisol, the fat-storing hormone, is released so it's better to have your big meal earlier in the day.

Perhaps it's no surprise that cutting back on sugary snacks will help heal adrenal fatigue. The body often craves sugary or salty foods in this state. Many people rely on caffeine to keep going, but overall this leads to a greater drop in energy. The best foods to support the adrenal glands with micronutrients are asparagus, avocado, garlic, cabbage and ginger.

3. TAKE SUPPLEMENTS

Vitamins B and C and omega-3 fish oils all support the adrenal glands. You could take these in the form of supplements, or eat more foods rich in vitamins B and C, such as avocados, grapefruits, strawberries, bananas, oranges and blueberries, to name but a few. Omega-3 fish oils are found in oily fish like mackerel and salmon. In addition, herbs such as ginseng, rhodiola, ashwagandha, timo cordyceps mycelium extract and L-theanine can all be helpful.

There are some herbal supplements that can help support the adrenal glands as well as a supplement with pituitary and adrenal concentrate from bovine source to aid the healthy functioning of the adrenal and pituitary glands, but this should be done under the supervision of a health-care professional.

4. EXERCISE, GENTLY

When you have adrenal fatigue over-exercising, such as a strenuous gym session, will only put more strain on the adrenals. It's more beneficial to do 15–30 minutes of gentle exercise a day. Walking, yoga and swimming are ideal forms of exercise. It's also good to get some fresh air whenever possible so ensure to walk outdoors.

5. MAKE TIME TO RELAX

Schedule some relaxation into your diary every day, even if it's only 5–10 minutes. Walking, hot baths, massages, reading and meditation are all simple but effective. Go out and have fun too. We relax when we are doing things we enjoy. Whenever you are stressed, take a few deep breaths through your nose. This helps to slow the heart rate down. We're all extraordinarily busy nowadays, but it pays to learn how to notice when we're first getting stressed, acknowledge it and take time out to have a cup of herbal tea or gather our thoughts. You will learn more about this in other chapters.

Did you know...

- 94 per cent of people wish they had more energy?
- Adrenal fatigue is a major cause of low energy but is not commonly recognised by conventional doctors?
- Adrenal fatigue could be the reason you can't lose weight?
- Fifteen minutes of gentle exercise a day is better for you than a strenuous gym session?

CHAPTER 5
DIGESTIVE HEALTH

The digestive tract is the largest organ in the body. It's essential for us to digest our food, absorb nutrients and remove waste and toxins. However, our digestive system also performs many other functions to maintain our health. A well-functioning digestive tract is necessary to provide vital nourishment and energy for the mind and body. Indeed, optimum function of the digestive system is essential for a resilient immune system and supports metabolic clearing and healing processes in the body.

Unfortunately, if your gut isn't functioning perfectly, you won't benefit from a detox or cleanse programme. So the first step before considering this is to get your gut balanced and healthy.

Below I list some of the most common gastric problems and how you can resolve them.

LEAKY GUT SYNDROME

This is a well-known phenomenon in the world of integrative medicine, but sadly not in conventional medicine. All I know is that when I treat patients for it, the symptoms they've had for years 'miraculously' disappear.

Ian is a 35-year-old consultant psychiatrist and a good friend of mine. We went out for dinner one night after not seeing each other for a while. He told me he'd been having a horrible time suffering with terrible acid reflux, abdominal pain and bloating. He'd seen his GP several times, and had blood tests, an abdominal ultrasound scan, even an endoscopy test, and they all came back normal, yet he was suffering with these horrible symptoms that were affecting his everyday life.

I wasn't surprised the tests were normal and I told him this. I knew what was wrong and how to treat it and I explained leaky gut syndrome in detail, starting him on an intensive supplement regime for three months. Within the first month his symptoms were nearly all gone, and after three months everything had fully resolved, with no dietary changes needed.

WHAT IS LEAKY GUT SYNDROME?

We all eat lots of different foods and when we do we produce stomach acid to break them down. The foods we were designed to eat, such as fruits, vegetables, poultry and other wholefoods, are quite easy to break down. But most, if not all, of us eat things we aren't really designed to digest, such as processed and fast foods, alcohol, coffee and fizzy drinks. As a result we produce more stomach acid to break these down which, over time, can damage the delicate lining of the stomach and gut. In turn, when we eat more such food we require more acid, which continues to damage the lining of the stomach and gut and it becomes a vicious cycle.

Consequently undigested food particles aren't absorbed properly and there is some thought that micro-particles pass through the gut undigested and pass into the body. When there are foreign particles in the body, the body mounts an immune response to destroy them. So white blood cells attack the foreign particles and the lining of the gut, causing even more damage. This causes pain, bloating and heartburn symptoms. Due to the constant attack the nutrients from food cannot be absorbed properly and this can lead to tiredness. It can also lead to weight gain as this attack causes bloating and swelling. The mainstay of treatment is to repair the lining of the gut with supplements. If you have leaky gut syndrome, a detox or cleanse will fail, because it doesn't matter how many good nutrients you put in your body, you won't be able to absorb them.

HOW TO TREAT LEAKY GUT SYNDROME

I use probiotics in the form of tablets with my patients to heal leaky gut, as well as improving many other symptoms and conditions which are outlined in more detail below. I also recommend the following supplements to heal the gut:

- *Digestive enzymes* – these help to break down proteins, peptides, carbohydrates, sugars, fats and lactose. These should be taken three times a day with meals to aid digestion.
- *Cinnamon* – soothing to the gut and helps stabilise blood sugars.
- *Caprylic acid* – a fatty acid that purges unwanted compounds from the gut. It's also very good at breaking down yeast or candida cells. The usual dose recommended is 1–2 grams three times a day with meals.
- *L-glutamine* – essential for the functioning of the small intestine. I recommend 3–5 grams a day.
- *Glucosamine* – a building block for connective tissues and helps to support the gut's mucosal lining.
- *Papaya concentrate* – papaya fruit is high in papain, a potent proteolytic enzyme that supports the breakdown of proteins. Papaya is also supportive of bowel function and has soothing effects on the stomach and the digestive tract.
- *Gamma oryzanol* – a natural extract of rice bran oil, which is soothing to the gut.
- *Garlic capsules* – contains allicin, a sulphur compound which may help to establish microbial balance.
- *Grapefruit seed extract* – may also support a healthy microbial balance in the gut.

There are good compounded makes of the above substances available that have the above ingredients in a capsule, which is the easiest way to take these nutrients as you then don't need to worry about doses and there are less tablets or capsules to take in this way. Over one to three months there is normally a marked improvement in symptoms.

PROBIOTICS

Our guts are full of good 'friendly' bacteria, which work to reduce dangerous bacteria from our food. They aid digestion and the absorption of nutrients. They also help peristalsis, which is the process by which food and waste moves through the digestive system. They protect our mucous membranes by stimulating the production of mucins, which are the proteins in mucous that lubricate and protect the inner layer of our tissues. They improve the balance of friendly bacteria in the genital area and reduce the chances of urine and vaginal infections. In the bowel, these bacteria help to produce essential B vitamins needed for the effective running of our neurological system and help you feel energised.

Our natural levels of these good bacteria can be reduced by a poor diet, stress, smoking, alcohol, hormone changes, surgery and medications. This is when a probiotic supplement could be needed.

Research has shown that probiotics could have benefits for conditions, from type 1 diabetes to fibromyalgia. Scientists are trying to develop specific probiotics to prevent dental cavities, probiotic lozenges for sore throats, probiotic nasal sprays and probiotic deodorants.[1]

Probiotic supplements come in many forms, but the ones most people know about are in the form of yoghurt or milk drinks that are widely available in supermarkets. These contain small amounts of 'friendly' bacteria but also contain sugar, dairy and flavouring. Probiotics also come in capsule form, which in general have higher levels and different strains than the drinks and yoghurts. If cost is an issue, taking a yoghurt or probiotic drink is still a good option.

You might need probiotics if you:

- suffer from heartburn, acid reflux or a hiatus hernia
- suffer from bloating
- get frequent colds
- feel fatigued
- have very smelly stools
- have a lot of wind
- suffer from allergies
- have IBS
- have constipation or diarrhoea
- have bad breath
- suffer from body odour
- have thrush, vaginal discharge or urinary infections
- have stomach pains
- take antibiotics more than once a year
- are prescribed statins, steroids, inhalers, or acid-suppressing stomach drugs

HOW PROBIOTICS CAN HELP YOU

As well as aiding abdominal symptoms such as bloating, pain, distension, diarrhoea and constipation, probiotics can help an array of other symptoms.

Colds and Flu

Probiotics can be of value in boosting a flagging immune system. Studies carried out on healthy people found that those who use probiotic supplements and probiotic foods have fewer colds and winter infections. Probiotics can prime the immune system and increase resistance to infection by producing antibiotics. Protect yourself by taking a daily multivitamin and a probiotic supplement, especially during the winter. Studies show that multinutrient supplements taken with probiotics for a three-month period can lessen the number and severity of symptoms and the duration of a cold by several days.[2]

Allergies

There is a link between bad gut bacteria and allergies. Studies are looking at whether probiotics might help asthma and allergy sufferers by switching off an inflammatory response in the intestine. Research shows people with allergies have lower levels of healthy gut flora.[3] Probiotics can help reset that bacteria balance, providing a protective barrier in the gut. Research also shows that people who include fermented milk in their diet have a better immunity to pollen (they have lower levels of an antibody that aggravates allergy symptoms).[4] They also had higher levels of the antibody IGG, which protects against allergic reactions. I advise taking probiotic supplements as they can ease the symptoms of respiratory allergies, such as asthma and eczema. It's important to remember that supplements can take between 12 to 16 weeks to work.

Bad Breath

Most body odours, such as bad breath, are caused by bad bacteria. Malodour can be caused by rotting teeth, unhealthy gums, poor digestion, the ulcer-causing bacteria *Helicobacter pylori* or any number of other illnesses. But the biggest problem is the bacteria in our mouths can feed on the almost constant supply of food that comes their way. Some people naturally have low numbers of bad (pathogenic) bacteria and far higher levels of protective bacteria in their mouths. Sadly, only 2 per cent of the population fall into this category and the rest of us have to work on rebalancing our bug population.

Dental Care

As well as practising good dental hygiene, boost your good gut bugs by adding fermented milk products, such as live yoghurt, to your diet. Take a probiotic supplement regularly. Such supplements work by reducing the risk of dental decay in children's teeth, meaning that fewer adult cavities develop later in life lessening the likelihood of mouth ulcers and other oral infections.

Tiredness

Do you ever feel tired after eating a meal? Taking a probiotic can help you digest a meal so that not so much of your energy is spent doing this. Probiotics also help you absorb nutrients better which in turn can be used to help you feel energised. Probiotics help remove waste and toxins from the body. When your body is full of toxins, your cells can't operate and are not getting the oxygen they need. This leads to pain, inflammation and fatigue. Probiotics have a cleansing effect and help eliminate built-up wastes from your intestines. When your body is clean on the inside and not bogged down with those wastes and toxins, your cells can get the oxygen they need. More oxygen means more energy for what you want to do.

YEAST/CANDIDA OVERGROWTH IN THE GUT

When you go to see most doctors, they're aware of thrush, or yeast overgrowth, in the mouth and in the genital regions, but rarely consider it in the gut. However, I've seen many patients suffering with this problem.

Take my good friend Vicky. Vicky and I have been friends since we were four years old and in terms of length of time, she is my oldest friend (in terms of age I was born the day before her so technically I'm the older one!). Vicky had been feeling unwell for some time. She was having lots of irritable bowel symptoms. Her stomach was swelling and getting bloated (she's normally very slim) and she was constantly feeling run-down and getting viruses. Vicky had been to see her doctor and was given medication to treat the symptoms, but the problem wasn't resolving itself and this was getting her down. She had some tests that showed candida over-growth, and went on a strict diet as well as taking supplements. This was several years ago and now she has made long-lasting changes to her diet and has since had no further problems.

WHAT IS CANDIDA?

Candida is a fungus and a form of yeast. A very small amount of it lives in your mouth and intestines. Its job is to aid diges-tion and nutrient absorption. However, when overproduced it adds to leaky gut syndrome by breaking down the intestinal wall and moving into the bloodstream, releasing by-products into the body and leading to various health problems, ranging from diges-tive issues to depression to tiredness.

CAUSES OF CANDIDA OVERGROWTH

Sometimes your gut isn't able to keep your candida levels in check and this causes overgrowth. The common causes for this are:

- a diet high in refined sugar and carbohydrates – sugar feeds the yeast
- living a high-stress lifestyle
- taking a course of antibiotics for a medical problem that also kills off the friendly bacteria in the gut

SYMPTOMS OF CANDIDA

The symptoms of candida are variable and some are listed below:

- skin and nail infections such as athlete's foot or toenail fungus
- feeling tired and worn down or suffering from chronic fatigue syndrome
- digestive symptoms like bloating, constipation or diarrhoea

- skin issues such as eczema, rashes, hives
- mood swings, anxiety and depression
- difficulty concentrating, poor memory, lack of focus, hyper-activity or brain fog
- vaginal infections, urinary tract infections, rectal or vaginal itching
- can contribute or worsen autoimmune disease such as rheu-matoid arthritis, multiple sclerosis or ulcerative colitis
- severe seasonal allergies and itching
- strong sugar and refined carbohydrate cravings

Candida is diagnosed based on symptoms and there are tests available to detect this too. A good functional medicine doctor who practises medicine as I do or a good nutritionist or naturo-path will be able to order and interpret these tests for you.

Treating candida fully can take up to six months and involves taking the measures mentioned above to treat leaky gut syndrome. It is also important to take a good probiotic as discussed on page 54. Changes in your diet are key to healing your gut. Sugar feeds yeast, so typically sufferers need a low carbohydrate diet and have to cut out sweets, chocolate, desserts, alcohol and flours. Cutting out refined sugar entirely and a reduction to just one serving a day of complex carbohydrates such as grains, beans, fruit, bread, pasta and potatoes will prevent candida from growing further and eventually cause it to die.

LIVER CLEANSE

The liver is the most important organ for naturally detoxi-fying our bodies. It performs vital roles in regulating, synthe-sising, storing, secreting, transforming and breaking down many different substances in the body. Some of these functions include regulating fat stores, cleansing the blood and removing waste products, neutralising and destroying toxins, manufacturing new proteins, breaking down alcohol, drugs and chemicals in the body, aiding the digestive process by producing bile, helping the body resist infections by producing immune factors, storing vitamins, minerals and sugars, maintaining hormone balance and controlling cholesterol.

It's important to note that the liver can become sluggish and function less than optimally due to high protein diets, too many refined carbohydrates, overeating, taking a lot of medication or drugs, alcohol, toxins and pesticides in our environment, chronic diseases such as hepatitis and lack of exercise. When our liver is sluggish and not functioning well it can contribute to us feeling sluggish and tired due to the build-up of toxins in the body. As such, I advise taking regular nutritional support to help your liver. There are many formulas on the market but look for ones that contain milk thistle, dandelion root, artichoke or beet leaf, and the herb Picrorhiza kurroa.

It's possible to do liver and gallbladder cleanses at home, but this is quite an intense process and I would only recommend doing this once you've already completed the three-week cleanse programme. If you're new to these sorts of techniques wait until your overall health and energy are improving, or speak to an integrative doctor or practitioner like myself for support. This liver/gallbladder flush aids an important detoxification procedure which will facilitate a clearing of the gallbladder – the liver reservoir to store bile which breaks down oil/fats.

The cleanse involves drinking apple juice with every meal for five days, and then taking a mixture of olive oil, lemon juice and Epsom salts to flush out the liver and gallstones. I've not given full instructions here as I feel this is best done with the knowledge of your integrative medical doctor or professional. There are many good online resources to learn more information and there is an excellent book by Andreas Moritz called *The Liver and Gallbladder Miracle Cleanse* (see Resources, page 239) that I have found very helpful for myself.

FOOD INTOLERANCES

In my opinion, most people have a mild gluten, wheat and dairy intolerance. Our body can cope with a small amount of these foods in our diet every now and again, but it wasn't meant to deal with these in large quantities. Yet the majority of us have dairy and gluten several times a day. These low-grade food intolerances lead to a build-up of symptoms such as abdominal discomfort or bloating, weight gain, poor concentration, aches and pains and, of course, tiredness.

Think about it, you may have a small quantity of milk daily in your tea, or have a piece of toast in the morning or sandwich for lunch. It all adds up. It also takes a lot of energy to digest these foods. My friend Temi told me that when she had a sandwich for lunch she felt very tired and sluggish in the afternoon, whereas if she had a salad she had more energy. The simple reason for this is that the body struggles to break down processed bread, but can cope well with foods that are easy to digest like salad and protein. Therefore I suggest to all my patients that they reduce the amount of gluten and dairy in their diet, and try to limit them to a maximum of five servings a week if they're having gastric symptoms, after an elimination period of at least three weeks where they restrict these completely.

It is important to understand this is not the same as a food allergy which would make you feel very sick or you have a strong allergic reaction if you eat a certain food. An intolerance means having too much of a certain food makes you feel sluggish, bloated and not at your optimum level of well-being and energy.

If you feel you have other food intolerances, or your gastric symptoms are not resolving with the guidance above, then there are many good food intolerance tests available if you want a full analysis to guide you further. Consult your holistic health practitioner for further advice.

You should now be aware that technically there's no such thing as irritable bowel syndrome. If you're experiencing symptoms, it's your body telling you that something is out of balance, and the symptoms won't go away until the balance in your gut is repaired and restored. In order to achieve true health and improve your energy, start with trying to fix what is going on in your gut. Use the guidelines above and the questionnaire on pages 12–18 to guide you. Once your gut health has improved you will notice changes such as not getting heartburn or bloating, that your bowels become more regular and even that you catch fewer coughs and colds and, best of all, bounce back from overindulgence quicker. This is the first step to improving your energy overall.

CHAPTER 6
BREAK YOUR SUGAR ADDICTION

During a recent interview I was asked what *one* change would make the biggest difference to an individual's health. It took me some time to come up with the answer, not least because so many things can improve our health. I thought about saying regular exercise, or having 10 portions of fruit and vegetables a day, or not smoking, but there was one that stood out above them all: cutting out sugar.

Believe me, I know this is a hard one. I love sweet things. If I didn't keep myself in check, I'd eat chocolate and cake all day every day and weigh about 20 stone. And this is with all my training and knowledge of health and nutrition. It's my cocaine and it's clear I'm not alone: in Britain the average person consumes 238 teaspoons of sugar *a week*![1]

We're buying fewer bags of sugar a year and consuming fewer calories from 'free' sugar like table sugar, fruit juice and honey, yet obesity continues to rise. Half of Britons are overweight and 26 per cent are obese, and this costs us £5.1 billion a year in health costs.[2] I correlate this to the rise in our sugar consumption, which is due to hidden sugar in our foods. Sugar is in everything: it's in all processed foods, including bread (even wholemeal), it's in our drinks, yoghurts and cooking sauces, to name just a few. But interestingly, there's no recommended daily allowance (RDA) for sugar, unlike fats, proteins and even vitamins and minerals. The amount of sugar we consume can contribute to our blood sugars fluctuating hugely, going from us feeling a massive 'high' to feeling extremely tired and lethargic once our sugar hit has worn off.

Are you addicted to sugar?

1. Do you struggle to walk past the sweet/chocolate/cake aisles at the supermarket without buying some?
2. Are there times you feel you *have* to have a sugar hit?
3. Do you have routines that revolve around sugar – like always having a pudding or chocolate at a certain time of day?
4. If you are forced to go without sugar for 24 hours do you get withdrawal symptoms like headaches or mood swings or feel lethargic?

If you answer yes to more than one of these questions then you may have a sugar addiction. Do not worry, this chapter is going to help you understand why this has happened and how you can break the addiction.

So where do these cravings come from? There are no poisonous foods containing fructose, which could explain why, in evolutionary terms, we are drawn to sweet foods. However, having a sweet orange or apple is hardly the same as having a slab of chocolate fudge cake or a bag of fizzy sweets. The introduction of high fructose corn syrups made the sweet taste easy to reproduce. Research from the USA shows when people have a diet which is 25 per cent sugar, there's a rise in LDL cholesterol and other markers of heart disease within just *two weeks*.[3]

The average diet

This is what an average person might eat in a day. The numbers beside each are the teaspoons of sugar (or equivalent) in each item – not added, but already in the product.

Breakfast: wheat-based cereal (2) with milk (1½), orange juice (5)

Lunch: chicken sandwich (3), bottle of cola (10½), chocolate bar (5½)

Snack: apple (3)

Dinner: glass of wine (1) ready meal (3)

TOTAL SUGAR INTAKE: 34½ teaspoons of sugar.

DAILY RECOMMENDED SUGAR INTAKE BY NUTRITION EXPERTS: 6 TEASPOONS FOR WOMEN; 9 TEASPOONS FOR MEN.

These are shocking figures. Even I was surprised when I saw it written down. However, it is important to know that sugar is added to our milk and even our bread and in nearly all ready meals.

Sugar is utterly addictive. MRI scans taken of people's brains while they eat it show that it is activating our brain in a similar way to cocaine. As the sweet substance hits our tongue, increased blood rushes to the brain, and dopamine is released as it would in response to drugs or alcohol. Research has also shown that people who frequently consume ice cream, cakes, chocolate or fizzy drinks build up their tolerance like drug addicts and alcoholics, so they have to eat more and more sugar to get the same satisfaction.

But sugar doesn't just make you fat and increase your chances of having a heart attack – if they weren't bad enough. Dr Lewis Cantley, a Harvard professor, advises that limiting sugar intake reduces the risk of cancer. This is because eating sugar spikes insulin levels which can cause adverse effects in other tissues in the body. In addition, cancer feeds on sugar. In fact, some tumours have their own insulin receptors and use sugar to grow. What's worse is they take it up before the other tissues and muscles in the body, so in effect cancers hijack the sugar from healthy organs. I think you'll agree, this is a lose-lose situation.[4]

SUGAR AND TIREDNESS

When we consume sugar it gives us a burst in energy that can last a few hours, but this is short-lived and we often experience a 'low' afterwards as the digestive system has to use a lot of energy to process these foods.

Sugar also disrupts the orexin system in our brain. Orexin is a protein-like molecule that regulates a wide range of mental processes, from sleepiness to hunger. People with very low orexin levels suffer from narcolepsy (the condition where you fall asleep unexpectedly all the time) and obesity. Studies have shown that injecting mice with orexin makes them more active and increases their metabolism, and low orexin levels makes people feel run-down and tired.

Sugar reduces orexin so we feel tired and therefore move less and do little exercise. Because we feel so tired we take more sugary foods for a little boost. Meanwhile our weight is increasing as a result. It's a vicious cycle. Conversely, a diet rich in proteins such as meats, fish and eggs excites orexin cells and turns them on, boosting our energy levels.[5]

HERE COMES THE SCIENCE BIT

Okay, so we know sugar is highly addictive and I think I've made it clear it's in *nearly everything* we eat. But why is this the case?

In the 1970s two vital publications, based on lengthy studies, were released. One of these – *Pure, White and Deadly* – is possibly more accurate than *The Celestine Prophecy*! In it, the writer – British nutritionist and psychologist, John Yudkin – predicts the obesity epidemic and the consequences of adding sugars to our diet long term. The second publication – the Seven Countries Study – showed that the populations of countries consuming the most fat also had the highest incidence of coronary artery disease.[6, 7]

This information in the Seven Countries Study was used by governments around the world to reduce fat in our diets. However, no one checked to see if these countries also consumed high levels of sugar. The study has since been criticised as the seven countries (from where the study takes its name) examined were picked by the author – and he did not include countries like the Netherlands, whose residents have a high-fat diet but a low rate of heart disease, or Chile with its low-fat diet but high rate of heart disease.

Following the publication of these studies, the food industries around the world fell over themselves to reduce fat from our diet. But when a processed meal is created without fat it tastes awful. So what do we have to add to improve the taste? Yes, you guessed it: the sweet stuff.

Most processed foods are also lacking in fibre. Fibre makes processed food harder to freeze, reduces the shelf life and lengthens the cooking time. But fibre is vital as it can prevent heart disease, diabetes, weight gain and some cancers, as well as improving digestive health. The role of fibre in balancing blood sugars, controlling weight and improving digestive health helps regulate energy in the body. With a diet high in sugar and low in fibre is it any wonder that we're in such a mess?

For decades we've heard, and believed, the inaccurate message that high fat causes heart disease and a range of health problems. The truth is, we're all on a lower-fat diet than 40 years ago, but we're all fatter and have higher rates of heart disease! In fact, recent research (from October 2013) shows that diets high in fat don't increase heart disease at all.[8]

Could it just be a coincidence that a lower-fat diet substituted with sugar is causing all these problems? No is the short answer.

Here is the long answer: glucose is good. It's the sugar used by the body to generate energy in every cell. When consumed, 80 per cent is usually used up by cells in the body and 20 per cent passes to the liver, where it is stored as glycogen for energy for the future. Glucose also turns off hunger by stimulating insulin and leptin – a hormone used to turn off our feelings of hunger and which also plays a key role in regulating energy intake and energy expenditure.

Fructose is the sugar used in most processed foods, fizzy drinks and sweeteners. It isn't used by the cells of our bodies for energy, so it all goes to the liver to be processed. It also doesn't turn off ghrelin, our hunger hormone, which is why some people can eat loads of cake and stop only after they feel sick. Fructose also doesn't stimulate insulin or leptin. In the liver, the fructose is turned into uric acid, the substance that at high levels causes gout. It also causes high blood pressure by blocking the enzyme that keeps blood pressure low. This is how fructose contributes to heart disease. It's then processed into fat – approximately 30 per cent of fructose consumed ends up as fat, which is why sugar, not fat, causes weight gain.

In terms of sugar being a poison, studies have shown it's processed in the same way by the liver as alcohol, and we all know *that* isn't good for you. Indeed, sugar causes eight out of the 12 problems that increased alcohol intake causes – high blood pressure, pancreatitis, liver dysfunction, obesity, heart disease, high cholesterol, addiction and it can pass to a fetus, but instead of causing fetal alcohol syndrome it causes fetal insulin resistance. This is why sugar is as addictive as alcohol, because the way the body recognises and deals with it is the same.

Strangely, we all know of the dangers of alcohol and smoking as there's so much health promotion around it, but there is much less promotion of the downside of sugar. Families have no idea how much harm they are causing themselves or their children by feeding them cola, sweets and cakes.

> ## Sugar: the bottom line
>
> Consuming large amounts of processed sugar causes spikes in our body's blood sugar. This causes a temporary surge in energy, but then causes a massive crash that leads us to feel more tired than we did to begin with. These constant highs and lows cause the body to stop being able to regulate our own energy. The bottom line: a diet rich in sugar is going to worsen any tiredness you already feel.

FRUIT

Of course, there is also fructose in fruit. So does this mean eating fruit causes the same problems outlined above? No. Let me explain why. A study showed that seven days of a high-fructose diet increases fat deposits in the liver and the muscles, as well as increasing triglycerides (the bad part of cholesterol) in the body and decreasing insulin sensitivity. The volunteers in the study drank a solution with 3.5 grams of fructose per kilogram of their weight.[9] If you weighed 70 kilograms, that means you would have to consume 245 grams of fructose a day to get similar negative effects. If you wanted to get this from bananas, you would have to eat about 35, or 20 apples, or 490 strawberries or 600 cherries. The point I am making is that it takes much bigger portions of fruit than we normally consume to create the negative effects that fructose causes, compared with the amount of fructose in cakes and fizzy drinks.

SWEETENERS

When I went to America as a teenager on holiday, I distinctly remember the label on the packet of a sweetener said 'this product could cause cancer'. I even saw this just a few months ago on a recent trip to California. In the 1970s, a study on laboratory rats showed an increase in bladder cancer due to consuming aspartame – a key sweetener. This has since been disproven by the Food and Drug Administration (FDA). However, many people still claim links between aspartame and headaches, cancers, fatigue and other neurological symptoms. This hasn't been proven either, but many of my patients experience an improvement in their symptoms when cutting out sweeteners.

More recent research has shown interesting results. The San Antonio Heart Study has shown that people who drink more than 21 diet drinks a week are twice as likely to become overweight or obese than people who don't drink them.[10] The problem with sugar and sweeteners is they can overstimulate sugar receptors, so it's possible you would find less intensely sweet foods like fruit not as appealing and vegetables practically repulsive. You may find you're more attracted to artificially flavoured foods with less nutritional value. The less nutritional foods you have the less vitamins and minerals you will be consuming and that will lead to an energy imbalance which can contribute to tiredness.

The Multiethnic Study of Atherosclerosis showed that a daily consumption of diet drinks was associated with a 36 per cent greater risk for metabolic syndrome and a 67 per cent increased risk for type 2 diabetes. Considering the purpose of these drinks is to reduce the risk of these conditions in the first place this is a sad state of affairs.[11]

Finally, sweeteners are as addictive as sugar. A study showed that when rats are exposed to cocaine, and then given a choice between cocaine and saccharin, most chose the saccharin.[12]

So What's a Gal (or Guy!) to Do?

Now you have all this knowledge will you completely stop eating sugar? I can already feel your resistance! Like me, you may find it a struggle. This is because of sugar's drug-like properties and the addictive way it affects our brain

This chapter is 'food for thought'. Weaning off sugar is a good idea but, as mentioned, it can be challenging. But don't worry, I'm here to help and I've created the energy cleanse plan, outlined in chapter 9, that will help rid you of your cravings.

Just remember that the sugar in an apple isn't the same as the sugar in a chocolate bar. An apple has sugar as well as nutrients, fibre and is low in glycaemic load, which means it won't increase the blood sugar and insulin levels in the same way as refined sugar. Refined sugar over time will also increase tiredness due to blood sugar spikes, cholesterol, inflammatory mediators and oxygen free radicals, and with them, the risk for diabetes, cardio-vascular disease and other chronic illnesses. So, make informed choices and try your best to make more good choices than bad and you will have already taken the first steps to breaking your sugar addiction.

A good place to start is by keeping a food diary for a few days and seeing how much sugar you really consume. Once you are aware of it you can try and cut down slowly. If you crave sugar and normally have a bar of chocolate every night, try and only have half instead. Replace sweet treats with healthier options like fruit with yoghurt. It is also important to consume lots of proteins like lean meat, fish, hummus and eggs and fats like coconut oil, avocados, nuts and seeds to help balance blood sugars in the body and curb cravings.

CHAPTER 7
CHEMICAL
NATION

Every day we are exposed to hundreds of chemicals: from pesticides that cover our fruit and vegetables to products we use to clean our house; from washing powders we clean our clothes with to the lotions and potions we put on our skin. But what does this mean and does it really matter?

What if I told you that *the biggest risk for getting diabetes is not how much food you eat and how fat you are, but how many chemicals are in your body?* And what if I also told you that these chemicals could also be the reason you are so tired all the time? Let me explain. Persistent organic pollutants (POPs) are organic compounds that are resistant to the environment and can accumulate in human and animal tissue. Examples of these can be found in pesticides, solvents, industrial chemicals, plasticisers and fragrances. Exposure can occur via many routes, such as through the skin and breathing them in, but a study showed that *diet* is the main route, causing more than 90 per cent of exposure in children and 80 per cent of exposure in adults.[1] An American study looked for 49 different POPs in adults and found at least 20 of them in more than 60 per cent of the US population. Worryingly, in those who had high levels of POPs in their body there was an increase in cardiovascular disease, high blood pressure, diabetes and obesity.[2, 3]

So, how do these POPs affect our bodies and cause symptoms and tiredness?

POPs have different chemical structures, but in general, they disrupt the endocrine system which makes hormones like thyroxine and our sex hormones. They interfere with insulin and affect the way the body can regulate blood sugar. On a cellular level they damage mitochondria, which the body needs to transport energy around the body, and inflammatory cytokines which are needed to fight infections and inflammation. They can also cross the placenta and affect unborn children. For example, one study showed that high umbilical cord blood levels of a POP called hexachlorobenzene are associated with a greater risk of obesity in children.[4]

As well as disrupting the thyroid gland, causing low libido and erectile dysfunction, POPs can cause hair loss, poor attention, memory loss, low mood and *fatigue*. When I first heard this I was surprised, but it made sense that the chemicals we're exposed to in our food and environment can contribute to feeling tired. No wonder there's such an epidemic, and it clearly isn't all our fault.

In adults, exposure to POPs is linked to diabetes, obesity, cardiovascular disease, inflammation and reproductive abnormalities.[5] A study showed a 38-fold risk of diabetes in those with the highest levels in six POPs. Due to the inability of the body to process blood sugars, tiredness is a major symptom of diabetes.[6]

There is some evidence that tiredness and fatigue are caused by low signals in the brain. This means that the neurons, which are the building blocks in the brain that transmit information, are functioning at a low level. This can be caused by low thyroid function, the adrenal glands not working sufficiently and causing high cortisol, and low DHEA hormone and sleep disruption. It can also be caused by exposure to heavy metals like lead, mercury, nickel and aluminium, cleaning solvents, pesticides and herbicides. Smoking, alcohol and high levels of caffeine with sugar can also cause neuronal hypo-excitability.

Does this really matter? I believe so. Three million people in the UK have diabetes, 20 per cent of adults have thyroid dysfunction, dementia is on the rise and we are a nation of tired people.

There is a whole range of very expensive tests that measure an individual's exposure to POPs.[7] A less expensive option is to measure an enzyme called gamma-glutamyltransferase, or GGT, which is a common blood test that most doctors can organise. This enzyme directly correlates to alcohol consumption, and is often high in alcoholics or regular social drinkers. Exposure to POPs induces GGT as a defence mechanism. Even within normal range, GGT predicts type 2 diabetes, gestational diabetes, coronary artery disease, hypertension, stroke, high cholesterol, fatty liver, chronic kidney disease and cancer. A normal range is usually below 50 units per litre (u/l). Men with GGT levels above 50 u/l have a 26-fold risk of diabetes compared to those with less than 10 u/l. Those with a level of 40–49 u/l, which is still considered normal, have a 20-fold risk. Levels which are high but still within normal range occur with obesity, environmental pollutants, cigarette smoking, excess alcohol, physical inactivity and a diet that is high in meat and low in fruit and vegetables.[8, 9, 10] Other tests that can be useful are to check the liver enzyme ALT (alanine

How to reduce the impact of POPs

Switching to organic fruit and vegetables and cutting down on processed foods is the main way to decrease your exposure to POPs (see chapters 8 and 9). The Children's Pesticide Exposure Study (CPES) in Seattle, USA showed that children having a normal diet had chemicals in their biological samples, but after five days of switching to an organic diet, they had much lower levels. This means that within five days of changing your lifestyle, the chemicals in your body can be much reduced.[11]

transaminase) and uric acid levels. Elevated levels of either of these can indicate high levels of POPs exposure.

So, now we know that chemical exposure, especially to POPs, is bad for us and causes a whole range of serious health conditions and fatigue, we need to know how to counteract this to regain health and energy. As well as reducing our exposure through food and the environment, we need to reduce the impact of it on our bodies.

Glutathione

Glutathione (pronounced gloot-a-thigh-own) is a very important molecule made up of amino acids, essential for staying healthy and preventing disease. It is a major antioxidant, important for immune function and to help the body self-detox. Glutathione can help reduce the damage done to the body by POPs. The good news is the body produces its own glutathione; the bad news is that poor diet, pollution, stress, toxins, medications, trauma, ageing, infections and radiation deplete our natural levels and production. Glutathione's power comes from the sulphur it contains. This sulphur acts as a magnet for all bad things in the body such as free radicals and toxins. The toxins in the body stick to glutathione, are carried into the bile and stools and then out of the body. Glutathione also recycles antioxidants like vitamins C and E in the body.

There are genes in the body that are involved in producing enzymes that create and recycle glutathione, however, they can become impaired for many reasons, including the chemicals and POPs we are exposed to. As we're exposed to more toxins than ever before it's a catch-22 situation. Glutathione is the most integral part of your body's detoxification system and when it becomes depleted it cannot remove toxins from the body as effi-ciently, if at all, and we can no longer protect ourselves from free radicals and infections. This can be the start of a downward spiral to chronic illness

As well as being essential for immune system functioning, detoxification and protecting our cells, glutathione is also essential for maintaining our energy metabolism.

At present, it is hard to find a supplement to take of glutathione as most are not well absorbed if taken by mouth, but there are many in development in the form of 'liposomal glutathione' as this is the best way for it to be absorbed orally. Unfortunately the ones I have tried taste of rotten eggs due to the sulphur in glutathione! Glutathione can be absorbed well nasally or through an infusion but there are few doctors that offer this service at present. Luckily there are many things we can do to boost this important molecule in the body.

How to optimise your glutathione levels and improve your energy

- **Eat sulphur-rich foods** such as garlic, onions and cruciferous vegetables like broccoli, cauliflower, kale and watercress.
- **Whey protein** is a great source of the amino acid cysteine, which is one of the building blocks of glutathione synthesis. 15mg twice a day is recommended.
- **Exercise boosts your glutathione levels** and also boosts your immune system, improves detoxification and enhances your own antioxidant defences. A combination of aerobic and weight-training exercises work best, for 20–30 minutes three times a week.
- **Taking glutathione supporting supplements such as alpha lipoic acid**, which is very important for energy production, blood sugar control, brain health and detoxification. The body makes it but it can often become depleted by stress. Take R-alpha lipoic acid 250mg twice a day. Unfortunately there are no studies

---

that advocate taking glutathione as a supplement to boost your levels. Instead you have to give your body the right ingredients to produce it.

- **Selenium** is an important mineral to help the body recycle and produce more glutathione. It is found in supplements and also in Brazil nuts.
- **Vitamins C and E** work together to recycle glutathione. Vitamin C should be given as a dose of 500mg a day and vitamin E 150iu daily.
- **Milk thistle (silymarin)** has long been used to boost the liver's functioning and will help boost glutathione levels. Take 100mg three times a day.
- **Folate and vitamins B6 and B12** are important for methylation, which helps the production and recycling of glutathione. Folic acid 1mg a day, vitamin B12 1mg a day and vitamin B6 50mg a day.
- **N-acetyl-cysteine** has uses in treating asthma and people with liver failure from drug overdoses. It can also be used to prevent kidney damage from dyes during X-rays. It has also been shown to improve bipolar disorder and high blood pressure. Taking this amino acid replenishes levels of glutathione. A dose of 300–1000mg daily is recommended.
- **A high ratio of omega-3 to omega-6 fatty acids** can protect against endothelial cell damage mediated by POPs.
- **Meditation and yoga** have both been shown to increase glutathione levels.
- **Studies have shown using a sauna** can help excrete heavy metals and chemicals through the skin, but mainly if used for extended periods of time such as one hour per day. Using an infra-red sauna has the best results. It is best to start with 15 minutes a day and build it up over time.

ACTION PLAN

If you live a healthy lifestyle but still feel tired, it could be chemicals that are causing your lack of energy. Think about the ways you can reduce chemical exposure in your own life and how you can improve your glutathione production to aid your body in its natural detoxification processes.

CHAPTER 8
FOOD FOR THOUGHT

I'm going to be honest with you and admit that taking a close, honest look at the foods you eat will be the toughest part of your journey to regaining energy. It may involve making a lot of changes to your lifestyle and diet, but I'm going to make it really manageable. Hopefully by now you will understand why these changes are essential to regenerate your energy and health for life, and not just as a quick fix.

We need to think of our bodies as having a bank balance in terms of energy. So, eating foods like vegetables and fruits, whole grains, nuts and seeds, organic white meat and fish, drinking fresh water, herbal and green teas, and exercising all contribute to the positive balance. Think of it as getting your payslip at the end of the month. Then as the month goes on, we smoke, drink and eat processed foods that are high in chemicals and sugars, and we don't move our bodies, so our bank balance slowly goes down until we fall into our overdraft, or negative balance.

The point of this section is to clear out that negative balance by cutting out the things that are bad for you and replenishing your body with the good stuff. And the best news is that this can be done in just *three weeks* by following the cleanse plan in the next chapter. Yes, you heard me right: all the damage going on in the body can be improved in just three weeks and you will *feel* better and more energised.

BODY ACIDIFICATION

It is thought that a number of health problems can be caused by acidity in the body. The body functions best when it's pH is 7.39, which is slightly alkaline. A normal range is from 7.36–7.42. A reading of lower or higher than these figures indicates acidosis (from 7.36–7) or alkalosis (7.42–8), meaning that the body can no longer function and illness appears.

The main causes of acidification are thought to be smoking and a diet that is rich in acidifying foods such as grains, alcohol, coffee, tea, refined sugars and processed foods, and low in alkalizing foods such as fruit and vegetables. Stress and either a lack or an excess of physical activity can also cause acidification. Following the three-week energy cleanse programme will help to restore balance in the body and alkalise it.

HIGH FIVE TO FIVE A DAY!

It's estimated that only one in 10 people in the UK eat the recommended 'five a day' portions of fruit and vegetables. This is rather worrying as in the USA and Australia the recommended portions are seven a day and in Japan it's 12 a day – so we're not even achieving the *lowest* recommendations. Very new research from April 2014 has shown that having '7 a day' can lower cardiovascular disease, cancer and death by any cause.[1]

The current guidelines are based on the World Health Organization's recommendations of ingesting 400g of fruit and vegetables a day to reduce the risk of serious health problems, such as obesity, heart disease, strokes and cancer. Therefore, five 80g portions of a variety of types and colours of fruit and vegetables are recommended, to ensure a broad range of nutrients, vitamins and minerals, as this varies across the different types.

Having your five a day can reduce the risk of cancer, especially bowel cancer. It also reduces your chance of getting heart disease

Do you have signs of acidification?

Find out with this checklist of 20 symptoms. If you have more than four of the below you could have body acidification.

1. Lack of energy or constant fatigue
2. Frequently feeling cold
3. Tendency to get infections
4. Loss of drive, joy and enthusiasm
5. Depressive tendencies
6. Nervousness, agitation without cause, hyperactivity, sensitivity to high-pitched noises and easily stressed
7. Headaches or migraines
8. Arthritis or rheumatism
9. Inflamed, sensitive gums
10. Mouth ulcers
11. Recurring infections of throat and tonsils
12. Excess stomach acid, acid regurgitation or gastritis
13. Skin tends to be irritated in regions where there are heavy concentrations of sweat such as under the armpits or the groin area
14. Hives or skin reactions and allergies
15. Leg cramps and spasms
16. A runny nose
17. Osteoporosis
18. Itching
19. Dull hair or hair falling out, and thin and split nails
20. Burning and irritation to the bladder or urethra

and strokes. Moreover, fruit and vegetables are our best source of vitamins and minerals which are essential for us to maintain good energy, and an excellent source of dietary fibre, so are very important in maintaining a healthy gut and stopping digestive problems and constipation.

Certain fruit and vegetables can help specific conditions. For example, if you are anaemic, beetroot can help stimulate red blood cell production and green vegetables such as spinach and other leafy greens are a rich source of iron which is needed for blood cell production.

Most people drink milk to get calcium, but did you know that leafy green vegetables, broccoli and peas contain more calcium (and in a form readily available to be used by our cells) than any dairy product?

If you have an underactive thyroid gland, iodine is important for manufacturing the thyroid hormones (see pages 36–7). Iodine is found in foods such as mushrooms, spinach and asparagus, and eating these can help support the thyroid gland.

These are just a few examples. There are many more I could use, but if I was going to list all the benefits of fruit and vegetables and all the conditions they can improve I would need a separate book!

The great news is that fruit and vegetables are very low in calories so you can eat more without gaining extra weight. The energy you get from fruit and vegetables is from carbohydrates and fibre rather than high calories. The sugars in fruit and vegetables are released and digested more slowly than those in a chocolate bar, therefore causing a sustained release of energy, rather than the high and low dips we get with sugary processed foods.

If cost is a concern, most of the UK supermarkets offer cheaper ranges of fruit and vegetables and many towns still have a local market where groceries can be bought at low cost. There are also low-cost shops where fruit and vegetables are often more affordable. Frozen fruit and vegetables are always a good option as the quality is good and most products are frozen quickly after picking so retain the nutritional value, and buying this is often more cost effective. To put the costs into perspective, market research showed that in 2008 we spent £3.5 billion on chocolate in the UK. If you go out for coffee once a day you'll spend £36,000 in your lifetime. The average Briton is now spending £1,320 on takeaway food every year. That's a lot of chips! All these foods are nutrition-ally barren and clog up our arteries and vessels. It's time to start thinking about spending your hard-earned money on foods that are going to give you some benefits, not cause you harm.[2, 3]

I've already used the car analogy in relation to the thyroid (see page 33), but it's also useful to compare your whole body to a car. When you own a car, you get it serviced and have a MOT regularly, you take it to the garage if it makes any noises or if a warning light goes on, and you make sure you fill it with the right fuel. However, we don't look at our bodies in the same way. We wouldn't dream of putting diesel in our car if unleaded petrol was recommended, yet we continue to put the wrong fuel into our bodies and not give them a regular 'service' but expect them to be fully functioning.

So while the best fuel for your body is fruit and vegetables it may seem overwhelming to eat so many of them. My suggestion for an easy way to get them in is to get a juicer and make fresh juices. I first heard about the benefits of juicing from a nutritionist who was a lecturer on my integrative medicine diploma course. She said she uses juicing with clients who have cancer or other chronic long-standing health conditions to help replenish and nourish the body. She found it particularly useful as an adjunct to help build the body back up, especially after harsh treatments like chemotherapy that destroy good and bad cells in the body and can have long-lasting effects from which the patient takes a long time to recover. Juicing is beneficial because you can drink more fruit and vegetables than you can eat, and drinking freshly made juice gives your digestive system a rest. If you juice 80 grams each of four different fruit or vegetables then that can count as four out of your five a day. What's more, the nutrients are easily absorbed to replenish the body quickly.

FOOD AND MOOD

As I've said previously, it's really important to become in tune with your body and understand the messages it sends you. Before I see a patient for a consultation, I ask them to fill out a food diary of everything they've consumed for three to four days and to record how they felt after each sitting. Certain foods can make us feel bloated or tired or energised. Let me give you an example. When I first saw Sara for a consultation, she was suffering from bloating, constipation and feeling really lethargic. We went through her food diary and it became obvious that when she ate dairy, yeast and wheat products her bloating was worse and it made her feel tired. We devised a new eating plan and after four weeks her bloating had gone, her bowel habit was regular, she had lost nine pounds in weight, felt energised and looked full of vitality. We were able to improve her condition in a short space of time and Sara didn't have to spend money on expensive food allergy tests. When you become the expert on you, you too will be able to see the clear link between what you eat and how you feel.

FOODS WE THINK ARE HEALTHY BUT ARE ACTUALLY NOT

Most people realise that eating large amounts of chocolate, chips and burgers is not healthy. But there are certain foods that people believe are healthy and are actually far from it. These are rather inconvenient truths, because if you're anything like me, once you know this stuff it will play at the back of your mind until you have to take action. Some people get angry with me for telling them, like I'm the one causing there to be pus cells in their milk… more on that in a minute! I'm just the messenger. What you do with this information is up to you, but at least you will be making an informed decision and not being duped by the food industry. Let's go through some of the key offenders.

MILK

I was brought up with the message that milk is good for you and needed to build strong and healthy bones. I was shocked when I found out the truth about milk and how it's produced. I first read about this in a book called *Skinny Bitch* by Kim Barnouin and Rory Freedman and have since done my own research confirming the facts by different sources including speaking to many farmers and vets.[4]

Firstly, we're the only mammals who consume milk after we're weaned, and also the only species that drinks milk from another species. It sounds very odd written out like that, doesn't it? However, the way milk is produced is my main issue.

In the olden days, you would get your milk from the local farmer who was able to supply the local community, but nowadays milk has to be mass produced to meet the demand to fill our supermarkets. For the supply to meet such demand, the cows have to be injected with hormones to keep them producing milk all year round, and these pass into our milk. The cows have to be milked constantly which leads to them getting mastitis, an infection in their udders. They're subsequently injected with antibiotics which also pass into our milk. The farms are more like factories, and the cows are often kept in cramped conditions with little living space. Infection is rife due to poor hygiene and unsanitary conditions. If that wasn't bad enough, the poor cows get such frequent infections that if we waited for them to fully clear up there would never be enough milk on our supermarket shelves, so our milk is allowed to have a certain amount of red and white pus cells in it. A litre of milk can contain up to 400 million pus cells. There are even some pus cells in some organic milk, but a lot less. Goat's milk is a better option but still has some infection cells. Moreover, cows with mastitis produce milk with less nutritional value, and dairy cows have their life expectancy reduced by 75 per cent. This is one of the many inconvenient truths about the modern-day food industry. It could explain why I see so many people with poor immune systems and hormonal problems.

Organic milk is a better option as the fats in it are healthier and there are few chemicals and antibiotics used. Cows are fed at least 60 per cent grass or hay, as opposed to a processed feed that most ordinary dairy-farmed cows get given, and no artificial fertilisers or herbicides are used. The cows also live longer and are less stressed as they can roam free and are not kept in pens. At present, a pint of organic milk is nine pence more expensive than ordinary milk.

I try to have as much soya, almond or rice milk as possible and reduce my intake of dairy products, or you could find a local farm shop and find out exactly what is going into the milk they produce and buy your dairy products from them.

There is some controversy about whether soya milk is good for you or not. The reasons for this are because soy is quite processed nowadays and also can convert to phytoestrogens and it is thought that it can interfere with our own natural hormones, but the evidence is not conclusive at the moment. I would advise women of child-bearing age to limit their soya intake, for example I only have soya milk if I am out in a coffee shop or a couple of times a week.

FISH

Fish is full of omega-3 fatty acids that protect the heart and is a good source of protein with less fat than meat and poultry. However, it also contains mercury and other environmental pollutants. The body can deal with a small amount, but children, women trying to get pregnant or those who are unwell should limit their amounts. Farmed fish should be limited as the nutritional value is lower than wild or organic fish, and their feeds are contaminated with chemicals, or they are fed other fish. It's also estimated that in North America, farmed fish have more antibiotics per pound in weight than any other livestock.[5] Farmed fish are also higher in fat than their wild counterparts. Farmed salmon is high in Poly Chlorinated Biphenyls (PCB) and dioxins, which are chemicals that drain our energy and affect our hormones.[6]

Wild or organic fish, on the other hand, have a diet rich in algae and other phytonutrients, so always choose wild or organic over farmed, and buy your fish from a reputable fishmonger.

WHEAT

Guess what? Bread and pasta aren't that good for you either. It's not so much that wheat is bad for you, but modern-day wheat and the way it's grown and processed is again the problem. Sixty per cent of wheat is processed into bleached white flour. Its nutritional value is degraded and over half of the B vitamins, vitamin E, fibre, calcium, zinc, copper, iron, phosphorus and folic acid are lost. Even in 100 per cent whole-wheat products, most modern strains are created by irradiation of wheat seeds and embryos with chemicals, gamma rays and high-dose X-rays to induce mutations.

People who have coeliac disease have an adverse reaction to gluten and need to avoid it entirely. If they don't, there will be ongoing gut symptoms and tiredness, and it could lead to osteoporosis (weak bones) and anaemia. However, I see lots of patients who don't have coeliac disease, but still suffer from tiredness and gut symptoms and feel much better when they stop, or reduce, wheat-based products. Wheat germ agglutinin (WGA) is a chemical in wheat responsible for many of the symptoms and ill effects caused by wheat.[7]

Should everyone cut out wheat? If you frequently experience abdominal pain, bloating, constipation, diarrhoea or excessive wind, then the answer may be yes, or at least try to cut down.

These symptoms are collectively known as irritable bowel syndrome (IBS), and are often caused by an inability to break down a group of sugars that naturally occur in food called Fermentable Oligo-, Di-, Mono-saccharides and Polyols, or FODMAPS.

If these sugars are not broken down in the small intestine, they travel on to the large intestine where they provide a free meal for your gut bacteria. These repay the favour by producing gas which leads to the bloating, pains, wind and the bowel changes often seen in IBS.

Studies, including the original study by SJ Shephard et al., have shown that avoiding FODMAPS – including fructan, the FODMAP found in wheat – can improve the symptoms of IBS.[8] People with IBS often find an improvement by avoiding high FODMAP foods such as avocados, cherries, apricots, nectarines, peaches and plums, honey, dairy, wheat, onions, garlic, lentils, beans and sweeteners.

Unlike those with wheat intolerance and allergies, people who may benefit from a low FODMAP diet do not have to completely avoid wheat (and other foods containing FODMAPs). They just have to acknowledge their symptoms will worsen with high FODMAP foods.

The simplest way to see if you're experiencing an intolerance to wheat is to simply cut it out of your life for two weeks. If you feel better, there's your answer. It's easy, quick and you don't need any expensive laboratory tests. After an initial period of cutting out the wheat, I normally advise my clients to restrict consumption to one or two times a week, and just a small amount at a time. I tell my patients to do the same with dairy if I think they're reacting to it, but not at the same time or we won't know which eliminated food product is making the difference. Remember, we weren't designed to eat food products like milk and wheat every day, and if we were, it wouldn't be the over-processed, chemically laden, pus-filled substances we're sold today. When we eat these products every day the body has to work hard to break down, digest and deal with them and never has a chance to carry out its other vital processes. By only eating these products a couple of times a week, your body has the ability to repair any damage done.

MEAT

If you are going to eat meat, try to eat organic or locally produced meat from a farmer or butcher. This is because non-organic meat can contain antibiotics and hormones as the animals are often fed food that has been treated with synthetic fertilisers, pesticides, herbicides, sewage sludge or radiation. Non-organic meat can be exposed to more chemical additives approved for use in food. Some meat producers inject their meat with additives to tenderise the meat, extend shelf life and add flavour.

If you need more convincing, watch the 2010 Oscar nominated documentary *Food, Inc.* to see how animals used for mass-produced milk and meat are treated, and the horrible conditions of the meat-processing factory. Be warned you may not want to eat meat again if you see it![9]

I'm not saying to cut all these foods out of your diet straight-away. To make long-lasting dietary changes is a process and it can take years to be in the right place physically, mentally and spiritually to make and sustain these changes. I became a vegetarian in my mid-twenties for three years (mainly because Russell Brand is a vegetarian and I'm a huge fan!). However, my decision wasn't based on my *own* values and mentally I just wasn't ready. Subsequently, I mainly ate chips, baked beans and cheese. I eat meat and fish again now, but very sparingly, and overall my diet is more balanced. I would like to be vegetarian in the future, but I know I need to embrace it in a spiritual way and really connect to my decision on a deeper level for it to be a successful, healthy and long-lasting change.

Someone once told me to avoid avoiding of foods. This means as soon as you make a food 'contraband' it suddenly becomes way more appealing! If you eat well and healthily the majority of the time, and every now and again want a fizzy drink or a burger, it isn't going to do you much harm. Remember the 70/30 rule, it is just all about balance.

I haven't told you the truth behind milk, meat and wheat

processing to scare you or make you feel bad about what you feed yourself and your family, I simply want to make you more aware of what is going on with the food industry, and to stop them from duping you into thinking you are feeding yourself well when they are really controlling what you give your family for dinner and tricking you into thinking they are healthy food. I think you deserve to know the facts and deserve to be treated with respect and be told the truth.

The first step is to process this information, which can take a while to get your head around. It's quite different to the messages we've received from the media and growing up. Then, make small changes and take it day by day. A good start is to try the energy cleanse in chapter 9 and see how it makes you feel. When you see and feel the difference in your body from making changes for just three weeks, you will feel more motivated to make long-lasting lifestyle changes.

'EATING CLEAN'

One of the key ways to increase energy and beat tiredness is to cut out chemicals. This means avoiding processed foods as much as possible. An easy rule is to think about how much human interference a food has had. For example, an apple is a wholefood, but an apple pie is flour, sugar, butter, etc., fashioned into food. Another example is that if a food has a long list of ingredients, a lot of which you don't recognise because they're additives, preservatives and other chemicals, it's best to avoid it. Whenever presented with a choice, try to pick the food that has been interfered with the least. This is what I try and apply to myself when I'm out and have to grab food on the go. If you do this you're on to a winner. I also try and keep snacks on me like dried fruit, seeds, nuts or healthy snack bars in my handbag so I don't feel starving and reach for a muffin. I call this *eating clean*.

ORGANIC FOOD

People always ask me if organic foods are really worth the extra money. Most people think that organic food means that no chemicals or pesticides are used. I did too for a while. Organic actually means 'fewer chemicals and a minimal amount of pesticides'. Because organic food is more expensive, the Environmental Working Group published guidelines on which fruit and vegetables should be eaten organic, and which ones are grown with fewer pesticides and can be eaten without being organic.[10] A study in 2012 stated that there was no benefit in eating organic food over non-organic food. The study stated that the nutritional difference between the two was not much, however, organic foods had 30 per cent less pesticides.[11] We know from chapter 7 that the less chemicals the better for our overall health, and this is reason enough for me to buy organic food wherever possible.

Foods that should be eaten organic:

- apples
- celery
- cherry tomatoes
- nectarines
- chilli peppers
- grapes
- cucumbers
- peaches
- potatoes
- spinach
- strawberries
- peppers
- kale
- courgettes

Clean foods that can be eaten non-organic:

- asparagus
- avocados
- cabbages
- melons
- sweetcorn
- sweet potatoes
- pineapples
- aubergines
- grapefruits
- kiwis
- mangos
- mushrooms
- onions
- papayas
- peas

If you really can't afford organic, then I recommend really thoroughly washing your fruit and vegetables to remove the chemicals used on them, and soaking them in water with white vinegar in a ratio of three parts water to one part vinegar for 15–20 minutes and then rinsing thoroughly before eating.

BUY LOCAL

Another passion of mine is buying local produce and shopping at farmers' markets. It's often cheaper than buying organic in a supermarket yet still really fresh as it hasn't travelled for thousands of miles. After a period of time you will be able to taste the difference between vegetables and fruit picked yesterday and those that have been factory-washed and sealed in plastic. I love buying local produce and supporting people from my local community. We're bombarded with news about the recession; well let's do something about it and give our money to the local greengrocer or butcher rather than a massive supermarket. If you go to your nearest supermarket, you'll be hard pushed to find local produce in there. Have a look next time.

It's also great for us to start eating seasonally. Local tomatoes taste much better than those that are artificially ripened with gas. Foods that are chilled, shipped and held in warehouses lose flavour every step of the way. When foods are harvested early to endure long-distance shipping, it won't have the full complement of nutrients either. It's also good not to eat something all year round; when you haven't eaten something for months, the deprivation leads to greater appreciation. Eating food shipped to your country from thousands of miles away creates a huge carbon footprint. By eating local food you can minimise your environmental impact. Even better, make a vegetable patch in your garden or get an allotment. The more connected we become with our food the better.

ALL CALORIES WERE NOT MADE EQUAL

How often have you heard someone say the key to weight loss is just to eat fewer calories and exercise more? After all, it's just a case of calories in, calories out.

To a certain extent this is true, but the fact is not all calories were made equal.

It turns out, some calories count more than others. There are 100 calories in a cookie and also 100 calories in a portion of broccoli. But there is a huge difference in how they affect your appetite, your energy levels and your long-term health.

A Harvard Study in 2012 showed that it is all about the quality of the calories not the quantity. To lose weight and be healthy, it is the source of the calories that is more important than the number of them. The study said that the kind of calories a person gets affects how efficiently people burn their energy, which is the key for losing weight and keeping it off.

The researchers took obese adults and got them to lose weight, and then try one of the three following diets to maintain the weight loss – the Atkins low-carbohydrate diet, a low-fat diet and the low-glycaemic index diet.

The results showed that a low-fat diet doesn't burn many calories compared to the Atkins or low-glycaemic index diet, and the low-fat diet also changed certain metabolic factors in the body that predicted weight gain.

The low-carbohydrate diet burned the most calories, but it also increased certain markers for stress and inflammation in the body, like the stress hormone cortisol and other risk factors for cardiovascular disease and other health problems.

The low-glycaemic index diet struck the right balance for the participants, helping dieters burn more calories, not as many as the low-carbohydrate diet, but it did not increase disease-causing stress markers in the body.[12]

When you eat healthy wholefoods that are not processed then you do not need to count calories, as the weight automatically comes off due to a range of internal metabolic processes. You will also feel much better in terms of your energy levels as your blood sugars will not be fluctuating as much.

HEALTH BENEFITS OF COFFEE

New research has shown that coffee is not all bad. It is extremely rich in a diverse group of antioxidants called flavonoids, which have anti-inflammatory, antiviral and blood-thinning effects. A study has shown that a cup of coffee a day can be linked to a 7 per cent reduction in type 2 diabetes risk.[13] A study has also shown that moderate coffee drinkers have a far lower incidence of abnormal liver function, liver cirrhosis and liver cancers.[14]

A report published in the *Journal of Alzheimer's Disease* demonstrated that people with high blood caffeine levels over the age of 65 developed Alzheimer's disease two to four years later than those with lower caffeine levels.[15]

As caffeine stimulates the adenosine receptors in the brain, it does energise and helps people to focus on tasks. Reaction time, attention and logical reasoning all improve.

Coffee acts as a mild antidepressant by aiding the production of neurotransmitters like serotonin, noradrenaline and dopamine and a study has shown that it could cut the risk of suicide in men and women by about 50 per cent.[16]

Other health claims are that caffeine makes people feel less stressed, happier and helps athletes perform better as it increases the amount of fatty acids in the bloodstream. This allows athletes' muscles to absorb and burn those fats for fuel, therefore saving the body's reserves of carbohydrates for later on in exercise.[17]

SO SHOULD CAFFEINE BE AVOIDED OR NOT?

The evidence is showing that one or two cups of coffee a day isn't necessarily bad for you and may have some good health benefits. However, if you are having more than this a day, then the addictive qualities may be coming into play. If you drink coffee I would recommend having it black because the protein in milk will bind to the coffee's flavonoids and reduce the anti-oxidant effects.

The health effects will be massively reduced too if you enjoy your coffee as a latte from a coffee shop as it will be full of sugar. But as part of a healthy lifestyle, one or two cups of coffee will convey the above health benefits and not cause side effects or addictive processes.

WHY DRINKING WATER
IS SO IMPORTANT

Go and drink a glass of water right now. The benefits to your health are much bigger than most people realise.

We can live for weeks without food, but only a few days without water. Our body is made up of 60–70 per cent water – therefore it makes sense that we need it to maintain good health. Blood is mostly water, and your muscles, lungs and brain all contain a lot of water. Your body needs water to regulate body temperature and to allow nutrients to travel to all your organs. Water also transports oxygen to your cells, removes waste and protects your joints and organs.

When the body does not receive a constant and reliable supply of fresh water, it has to ration what is available and cut back on certain functions in order to make the supply go further. Essential systems like the brain are prioritised, while others are impaired or cut back until the brain has had its needs met. Other signs of mild dehydration include chronic pains in joints and muscles, lower back pain, headaches and constipation. Constipation is a definite sign of dehydration, as the intestines extract every precious drop of water from your food, to save losing it, creating a gridlock.

Another sure sign of lack of water in the body is a strong odour to your urine, along with a dark yellow or amber colour. Patients often come to see me with these problems thinking they have a water infection when they are just very dehydrated. Thirst is an obvious sign of dehydration and in fact, you need water long before you feel thirsty.

In most of us, the thirst mechanism is so weak that it is often mistaken for hunger. Even mild dehydration can slow down your metabolism. So if you are looking to lose weight, water is your friend. A study published by the *Journal of the American Dietetic Association* in 2008 found that drinking a glass of water before a meal resulted in a 14 per cent decrease in food consumption.[18] Do not fill up on fizzy drinks and shop-bought juices that are full of sugar and empty calories. If you find the taste of water boring, flavour it with some slices of fresh oranges, lemons, limes or watermelon or even some berries to make it more interesting.

Dehydration can trigger fuzzy short-term memory, headaches, difficulty focusing on the computer screen or on a printed page. And guess what? A lack of water can also cause you to feel tired.

Most of us have become chronically dehydrated, especially the elderly. Most people have decided that water is too bland to drink and instead replace it with tea, coffee, beer, wine, fizzy drink, flavoured water and other chemical-laced water alternatives. These alternatives do not hydrate the body, as many have a dehydrating effect because of their chemical composition.

Save money on Botox, just drink water

Your skin is the last place that water goes to, as it is low on the list of the body's priorities to hydrate compared to the brain and other internal organs. Therefore your skin is a reflection of your internal body health. If your skin is very dry and flaky, you don't need a good moisturising cream, you need to drink a lot more water. Because if your skin is in that condition – imagine what your internal organs are looking like!

Wrinkles and other facial lines are far less noticeable when the skin is well hydrated. So you can save money on expensive face creams and drink more water!

Do you want to get rid of your cellulite? Drink more water! Hydrated skin shows the dimpled skin less so the underlying fat cells are less noticeable.

Your eyes are made up of 92 per cent water, therefore to get brighter and more sparkly eyes, get drinking more H_2O!

I recommend my clients drink at least one and a half to two litres of water a day for optimum health and hydration; this is between six to eight glasses. Sparkling water is a good choice too, for even though it is carbonated you still get the beneficial hydrating effects. Of course this requirement goes up if you are in a warm country.

Drinking water isn't the only way to reap its health benefits. Zen Buddhist monks have incorporated water features in their meditative gardens for hundreds of years because of the soothing sounds. Studies have also shown that listening to the sounds of running water in nature or waves of the sea help to reduce anxiety.

Fruit and vegetables are made of up to 80 per cent water, so you can hydrate by drinking fresh juices or eating them raw and get your vitamins at the same time. A study from Japan showed that women who hydrated by eating fruit and vegetables had lower BMIs and smaller waists than those who just drank water. Watermelons are 92 per cent water, peaches 88 per cent and cucumber 96 per cent.

I've shared a lot of information in this chapter and I understand it can be overwhelming. Take some time to absorb the information and see if there are any small changes you can make right now. Don't be hard on yourself and don't try to do too much at once. I'm on this journey with you and know how hard it is to make changes, but you can do it!

The next chapter goes through the three-week energy cleanse in detail so that will give you a great kick-start.

CHAPTER 9
THE TIREDNESS CURE THREE-WEEK ENERGY CLEANSE

The three-week energy cleanse is designed for people with busy lives who don't have a week to go and only drink juice at a retreat. I've been on juicing retreats and felt amazing afterwards. Being away from my usual temptations, surrounded by people who are only juicing and not eating, lying in the sun and doing regular yoga has really been beneficial to me. However, I understand it can be difficult to do that even once a year due to our busy schedules and expense. However, there is no point in being mega-good for one week of the year and eating junk food for the other 51.

So, I designed this three-week cleanse for busy people who want to feel more energetic, less tired, eat healthily, but also want to retain some flexibility. If you have a dinner booked you won't need to cancel it on this programme as I'll give you the healthiest options to choose. I want to make healthy choices as easy as possible, because if it's easy, there's more chance you will stick to it.

This three-week cleanse will make you feel better than ever by gently weaning you off sugar and resetting your metabolic balance. It will help you regain your energy and vitality, lose weight and feel confident and fabulous. I've tried loads of detox and weight-loss plans throughout my life and I've taken the best of all of them and put them into my three-week cleanse. Based on my experiences, I honestly believe this is the easiest plan to follow without having to hibernate for three weeks and give up work and your social life.

People often presume a detox is just about what they eat and put into their bodies, but it's also important to cleanse your mind, use good natural products on your skin which contain few or no chemicals and let go of negative emotions in order to really restore your energy.

Another good reason to do a detox or cleanse programme at least twice a year is to give the digestive system a rest. Did you know that our digestive system produces as much serotonin, the happy chemical, as our brain does?[1] Therefore a sluggish gut can affect our mood, mental well-being and energy levels. When our digestive system is in good health, it absorbs nutrients and removes toxins more effectively. Just like the skin on our bodies is shed and regenerated every few months, so is the lining of our digestive system. A detox allows the lining to recover and regenerate from the stresses caused by the foods, drink, chemicals and drugs we consume.

So how does it work? Week one is an induction week, where you very gently reduce your bad habits, choosing instead unprocessed foods and fruits and vegetables. In weeks two and three we add in more liquid meals and supplements for a deeper cleanse.

THE HISTORY OF DETOX

The principles of detoxification aren't new. In fact, they originate from the ancient Egyptian and Greek ideas of autointoxication, which acknowledged that some foods can cause toxins harmful to the body. Every religion promotes fasting, from Judaism, Hinduism, Islam and Christianity, and is traditionally associated with penitence and purification. As such it has played a part in various cultures for over a thousand years.

However, as yet, no scientific evidence has proven that detox diets are effective, therefore some scientists have declared we don't need to detox or cleanse the body as it has methods of cleansing itself. This is true in principle. The body has processes for removing toxins through sweat and faeces and the lymphatic system, but in our modern times these can become less effective due to being exposed to chemicals through pesticides and preservatives in our food, pollution and drugs, the excesses of food and alcohol we consume, and our busy lifestyles.

Recent research showed that having two days of fasting a week is very beneficial to your health. As well as contributing to weight loss, having two days a week of 500 calories for women or 600 calories for men has been shown to regulate your blood sugar, which can lead to improved energy levels, and can also be protective against heart disease and illness.[2]

My experiences with my clients – and myself – have shown time and time again that detoxes are incredibly beneficial for allowing the system to rest and recharge.

My experience as an integrative medical doctor is that most illness is caused by chronic inflammation in the body, and this inflammation is mainly caused by the foods we eat as well as high levels of stress. Research has shown that inflammation is a contributing factor to cancer, heart disease and Alzheimer's disease. A cleanse programme is a good kick-start for reducing inflammation and introducing a healthier way of life and eating.[3, 4, 5]

Therefore I invite you to join me on a three-week detoxification cleansing process to kick-start a new period of healthy eating, to support your body while withdrawing from caffeine and sugar and to replenish your energy.

WEIGHT

The primary aim of this cleanse is not to lose weight, but my clients always do because they've made significant dietary changes and, in some cases, are doing more exercise than usual. If weight loss is important to you then weigh yourself before and after the programme. You can also measure your waist and see if that reduces. Often when I'm exercising I don't lose weight in kilograms but my shape changes and my waist size decreases.

BE PREPARED

Preparation is the name of the game. Quite often I work for several days in a row from 9 a.m. until midnight. This means I need to be super-prepared in order to make healthier choices and so I'm not tempted to grab a burger and chips on the way home from the night shift.

A word of advice: the more preparation you do, the easier this will be. First of all, get rid of temptation! Dump all processed foods, potatoes, pasta, bread, cake, desserts, chocolates, crisps, junk foods, fizzy drinks, tea, coffee and milk from your house. My weaknesses are chocolate and cake so I have to remove them before I do a cleanse plan. If you're worried about wasting food, why not donate the items to a food bank, or give them to a charity or a shelter or someone who you know would enjoy these foods?

Next, try to choose a three-week period where you don't have any social occasions so you can more easily avoid alcohol and overeating. If you like, have a 'final meal' of processed foods, desserts, etc. if you think it will help you psychologically before you start this process.

Some people find it's worthwhile doing a shop to get everything you need once a week. This cuts down on the temptation to buy unhealthy foods. Some like the flexibility of buying what they need every few days so that they do not over-buy and waste food, especially as fruit and vegetables can go bad if not used within a few days. Other people spend some time planning their meals for the whole week and then only buy exactly what they need. Do what works best for you, but whatever way you do this, the aim is to replenish your house with healthy foods.

Use the list below as a guide. You do not have to get everything on the list, but it is an indication for what you can eat during the plan. You do not have to buy anything you don't like, but it's sometimes good to try new things.

Good nutrition is how we absorb sunlight and energise our bodies. When we think about what we put into our bodies in that way, you can see why the list below is full of delicious nutritious foods to help us connect with the earth and sunlight and feed our own natural source of energy.

SHOPPING LIST

This is a very basic shopping list to help you on your way:

- Chicken: breast, legs, drumsticks, any type is fine, skinless is preferable
- White fish: cod, squid, scallops
- Tuna
- Oily fish: salmon, mackerel, herring, sardines, anchovies
- Turkey
- Prawns
- Mussels
- Vegetables – anything you like. Try and get a variety of colours, for example red cabbage, beetroot, carrots, red peppers, as well as the usual green broccoli, spinach, etc. Other suggestions: brassicas – broccoli, cauliflower, Brussels sprouts, cabbage. Dark green leaves: kale, rocket, lambs

lettuce, spring greens, tomatoes, cucumber, asparagus, green beans, mushrooms. Root vegetables: parsnips, pumpkin, swede, butternut squash, sweet potatoes

- Salad – pre-prepared mixed salad is fine
- Eggs
- Couscous
- Brown rice
- Rice noodles
- Lentils
- Chickpeas, butter beans, adzuki beans (also known as aduki and azuki), kidney beans
- Hummus
- Fruit (all)
- Oats (porridge)
- Sugar-free muesli
- Rye bread
- Non-dairy milk: soya, rice, almond
- Nuts: almond, Brazil, walnuts (unsalted)
- Seeds: pumpkin, linseed, flaxseed, sunflower
- Dried fruit
- Olives
- Nut butters
- Herbs
- Spices
- Olive oil/flaxseed oil
- Coconut oil
- Balsamic vinegar
- Herbal teas
- Still mineral water
- Protein powder for shakes: there are many good brands on the market which are flavoured and full of vitamins and minerals, or you can buy plain whey or hemp powder from a health-food shop and add your own fruit or flavourings.

Make sure that the brand you use has approximately 20g of protein per serving.

- Healthy snack bars. These are available from most health-food shops. Be sure to check and make sure there are no added sugars.

FOODS TO AVOID

- No dairy products. This includes milk, cheese, cream, yoghurt
- No alcohol
- No coffee/tea
- No white potatoes
- No white pasta
- No white rice
- No chocolate/cakes
- No wheat
- No processed foods
- No added sugar

HONEY

You may notice in some of the recipes honey is included in the ingredients. If it is possible, use a high quality honey like Manuka honey, but if this isn't possible within your budget a small amount of regular runny honey can be used in the recipes. If you have a sweet tooth and are missing sugar, the ideal sweetener would be a small amount of a fruit based sweetener like stevia.

HOW TO COOK

The main ways of cooking during this programme are as follows: grill, poach, steam, bake, lightly frying in coconut oil or olive oil and stir-fry. These are healthy ways of cooking that do not use excessive oil. Frying should be avoided during the three weeks.

A lot of people nowadays cook with their microwave. If you want to do this, avoid microwaving or over-boiling your vegetables. One study showed that microwaving broccoli at 1000W in a lot of water reduces nutrients by up to 97 per cent. Steaming in general only reduces nutrients by 11 per cent.[2] However, if you microwave vegetables with only one to two teaspoons of water in a sealed container it reduces the nutritional depletion.[3]

SELF-ASSESSMENT OF YOUR CURRENT ENERGY

It is difficult for health-care professionals to measure fatigue as it's such a subjective symptom. There are some scales, such as the Piper Fatigue Scale, which have shown reliability and validity when tested.[4] It is sometimes hard to judge how you feel when doing a programme and by assessing how you feel before and after the three-week cleanse will help you clearly see and understand the changes you have experienced.

Below is a self-assessment that you can do before you start the programme and then after if you would like to see how much you have improved. There is a link on www.holistic-doctor.co.uk for you to download a copy if you prefer.

For each of the following questions, score yourself out of 10 for the response that best describes the fatigue you're experiencing currently.

1. How severe do you feel the fatigue you currently have is?
    Not at all   **Very debilitating**
    1   2   3   4   5   6   7   8   9   10

2. To what degree is the fatigue you are feeling now interfering with your ability to complete your work – i.e. do you ever call in sick or put off work due to tiredness?
    None   **A great deal**
    1   2   3   4   5   6   7   8   9   10

3. To what degree is the tiredness you are feeling interfering with your ability to socialise – i.e. do you ever cancel plans or opt to stay in due to fatigue?

None   **A great deal**
1   2   3   4   5   6   7   8   9   10

4. How much do you rely on stimulants like caffeine or sugar to keep you going?

Never   **Many times on every day**
1   2   3   4   5   6   7   8   9   10

5. Do you think that the fatigue you are experiencing is:

Normal   **Abnormal**
1   2   3   4   5   6   7   8   9   10

6. To what degree are you now physically feeling:

Strong   **Weak**
1   2   3   4   5   6   7   8   9   10

7. On the scale of 1–10, how would you describe your stress levels?

Relaxed   **Stressed**
1   2   3   4   5   6   7   8   9   10

8. On the scale of 1–10, how do you feel?

Able to think clearly   **Unable to think clearly**
1   2   3   4   5   6   7   8   9   10

9. Would you describe your mood as:

Happy   **Depressed**
1   2   3   4   5   6   7   8   9   10

Add up your scores and see what your total is out of 90. You can then repeat this at the end of each week of the cleanse or just at the end of the whole cleanse to have an objective measure of how much your energy has improved.

Alexis's Experience

It can be daunting when starting a new programme for your health and wellness, so here are some words of inspiration from one of my first 'cleansers', the lovely Alexis:

I have struggled with my weight for many years and am what you would call a 'yo-yo dieter'. You name it, I've tried it – every single diet has led me to feel deprived and eventually go on a binge that ruined all my hard work. I felt sluggish, bloated and, quite frankly, FAT all the time. As well as this I was always tired and never had the motivation or energy to do anything in terms of exercise.

Since starting this plan, I have felt healthier in general, my skin is fresher and smoother, meaning I am using less make-up to cover up blotchy/dry patches as they no longer exist, friends and family have also commented that my skin is 'glowing' since doing the plan. People are seeing me enjoy the plan and can see outward signs of my success so are even saying they will make changes to their own diets to try to get the same effects. I have more energy now than I have had for as long as I can remember and actually WANT to go out and exercise 4–5 times a week.

I now crave fruits, nuts and seeds instead of chocolate, crisps and bread and have even experienced my first night/meal out without alcohol and didn't miss it at all.

– Alexis Hare, Cardiff, UK

Now you have assessed your energy levels and filled your cupboard and fridge with all sorts of lovely, healthy food, it's time to start the cleanse. I hope you're excited! This is the very first step to feeling less tired and more energetic, less run-down and more vibrant, less sluggish and more ready to take on the world!

WEEK ONE: INTRODUCTION WEEK

Week one is all about resetting your body and reducing your cravings. This will be easier if you have support around you, which is why slimming clubs work. With the weekly accountability and weigh-in you feel more compelled to stick at it as it is difficult to justify why you haven't met your targets and goals.

Sometimes, when you make changes in life, you come across resistance from others who – for whatever reason of their own – want you to stay the same way. I certainly know from my own experience that people say things like, 'Why do you want to do that?' or 'Isn't it dangerous?' They may be well intentioned but it's easy to let that put you off. People often want you to justify why you are eating well, so you can say you've been under the weather and need to eat better, or make out you are really not enjoying it, as people seem to find it more acceptable if you are on 'a diet' and hating it. If you are up to it you can just be honest and tell people what you are doing and why. You never know, you might inspire them!

It's really good if you can call on a friend to support you. Perhaps you could do the three-week cleanse together? Also, make sure that your partner is on board. He or she may not be ready to change his or her diet, but if they can support you in your choices – perhaps making their own or the children's lunches and dinners – then you'll be more likely to successfully complete the three-week cleanse. Some of my clients have told me their partners 'eat clean' in the house with them to support them, but then eat as they please outside the home when they are not there so my client can avoid the temptation.

I have an online community for my clients who do my cleanse programme so they can share recipes and support each other. Some of these people have never met each other, but receive support and can often share more with strangers than with their own families.

WEEK ONE: EATING PLAN

The first week is a gentle induction to wean yourself off your old unhealthy diet and cravings. We are aiming to avoid you being hungry and then making an unhealthy eating choice.

For lunch and dinner, I find it best to divide an average sized dinner plate into four quarters and fill it as follows: half with vegetables or salad, a quarter with protein and a quarter with carbohydrates such as brown rice or couscous or sweet potatoes.

I recommend having a breakfast high in protein, as studies have shown that this boosts your energy, helps you burn fat throughout the day and keeps you fuller for longer. In fact, it is important to have some protein with every meal to boost energy levels and keep hunger at bay.

WEEK ONE: THE WEANING-DOWN PROCESS

The two things people struggle with the most is detoxifying from caffeine and sugar. If you're really struggling without coffee, instead of giving up I recommend having a diluted cup made with half your usual amount of coffee, and cut it down by a cup a day. If you want to use decaffeinated for a few days that is also acceptable. The withdrawal effects normally only last two to three days so if you can cut it out completely and go 'cold turkey' that would be even better. Green tea also contains caffeine but has added health benefits, such as increasing metabolism and having antioxidant properties, so can be used as a healthy substitute.

If you're struggling with sugar cravings, take an amino acid supplement called L-glutamine. Glutamine can be taken in one capsule of 500mg up to once an hour, and if taken on an empty stomach can trick the body into thinking it has sugar in its system. It's safe to take and not known to cause harmful side effects. People who are low in chromium often suffer from sugar cravings, so it could also be worthwhile taking a supplement of this. There is another supplement called caprylic acid, which can help stabilise the blood sugar. It's a component of coconut oil, and is thought to reduce sugar cravings when on a low-sugar diet. It can be taken in supplement form at a dose of 350mg a day.

This 'weaning-down' process will mean that by week two you will be free of caffeine and sugar and feeling good.

Sample daily menu

Breakfast

Choose from:

- juice or smoothie with some nuts
- porridge made with non-dairy milk with added nuts and seeds and a banana or some honey or agave syrup to sweeten
- scrambled eggs with smoked salmon or turkey rashers
- omelette with some meat or vegetarian sausages for protein

Snack

Choose from:

- handful of nuts and seeds
- trail mix (see page 143 for recipe)
- hummus and carrot sticks

Lunch

Divide your plate into four and make sure it consists of the following:

- a half plate of salad or vegetables
- a quarter plate of protein of your choice such as chicken, hummus, tuna
- a quarter plate of carbohydrates such as couscous, brown rice or sweet potato

Snack

- snack bar, piece of fruit

Dinner

As for lunch, divide your plate into four:

- a half plate of vegetables
- a quarter plate of carbohydrates
- a quarter plate of protein of your choice

If this is a totally different way of eating for you and you feel like it is going to be a real challenge, why don't you start by 'eating clean' for two days a week and gradually build it up to more days over a few weeks. You will still experience benefits and notice an improvement in your health and energy. If you have children it would be completely safe and beneficial for them to 'eat clean' for a few days a week too.

WEEK ONE: EATING OUT

Another difficulty that people experience is what to do if they are out and about and have to buy food. This doesn't have to be hard. Most well-known coffee-shop chains sell reasonably healthy salads nowadays, and if you are out for dinner you can order a salad. I often order a fish or chicken dish with vegetables, and just avoid the chips. If you have to pop into a supermarket, you can pick up some cold meat or hummus to go with a pre-prepared salad pack. To avoid being 'caught short' if there really is no healthy food available, I try and keep a banana in my handbag or some healthy snack bars or a bag of mixed nuts, seeds and dried fruit. That way I really don't have a good excuse for grabbing a bag of salt and vinegar crisps!

WEEK ONE: OTHER ADVICE

I recommend eating as much raw food as possible during this time. This is because raw fruits, vegetables, seeds and nuts will help detoxify the body even quicker. The benefits of incorporating raw foods into your diet is that you will intake more enzymes, vitamins, minerals and phytonutrients than if all your food is cooked. The enzymes in food help convert it into a form the digestive tract can process, but also help energy, have anti-inflammatory effects, help boost the immune system and aid repair in the body. When we cook food we destroy many of the enzymes that help us naturally digest it. I would try and have some raw food with every meal, in the forms of smoothies, juices or salads

Top tips for eating out:

- Check the menu in advance and plan your meal
- If there's nothing suitable try and change the venue or call the restaurant to ask if they can work around your dietary requirements
- Take your car so you won't be tempted to give into drinking alcohol
- In most restaurants you can go for a salad option, or a meat and veg option
- In an Indian restaurant try and go for a dry chicken dish like tikka with dhal or plain rice and veg
- Chinese and Thai are tricky! But look for a stir-fried rice or noodle option and they always have soups. Thai restaurants often have salad. Avoid sauces as they are full of calories
- Eat well all day before you go out so you feel less hungry and don't end up feeling like pigging out
- Drink a pint of water before you go out. We often mistake thirst for hunger
- Before you go out, remind yourself why you started this plan. Keep motivated. This is your choice and it's not for ever
- Try to only go out with supportive friends who won't try and force you to eat cake for dessert
- If you slip up don't punish yourself. Just dust yourself off and start again. And be extra 'good' for a couple of days!

There are specific ways of making completely raw-food meals and you can look for classes in your area. You can also look to buy or make really delicious and nutritious chocolate mousse, brownies and other desserts if you have a sweet tooth (see pages 142–3).

I don't recommend taking any other supplements at this stage as your body will be dealing with enough changes as it is. It's common to have a bit of a headache or feel slightly fatigued for the first two to three days, so again, if you do this on days where you aren't too busy that might make it easier for you. If you need to sleep a lot you should allow yourself to do this for the first few days, as your body needs sleep to repair damaged cells. If you are on prescription medication you should continue to take this, but avoid any unnecessary over-the-counter medications. If you smoke, cutting out the cigarettes would also be hugely beneficial and you must try your best to avoid alcohol during this period.

Exercise is also helpful at this stage, but avoid intensive workouts and focus on more gentle exercise that is restorative for the body and soul, especially for the first few days, such as yoga, Pilates, swimming or walking. A good start would be a 15- to 30-minute session which you can build up over time. I recommend walking outside as much as possible for at least 20 to 30 minutes.

Relaxation is also important. As I mentioned previously, stress is toxic to your body and sets up inflammatory processes, so it's important to spend time relaxing every day. That can include meditation, practising mindfulness, going for a walk, listening to your favourite music, reading a book or writing in a journal. I would recommend 15 minutes a day at this stage.

Affirmations are phrases you repeat throughout the day that are meaningful to you. They're useful for keeping you motivated and to challenge any limiting beliefs you may have about yourself and life in general. Useful ones for this programme include:

'I am committed to improving my health and energy'
'I love and value myself'
'I feel strong, healthy and full of energy'
'I am vibrant and full of vitality'
'I am taking steps to improve my energy'

'Every day I am moving towards the life I want and deserve'
'I deserve a fantastic life'
'Every step I take, I feel stronger and more energised'

Use the ones that resonate with you or you can create your own. Write them down 21 times and also say them out loud 21 times. You can also say them in your mind if you're in public, or use them in your meditation as a mantra to focus on.

Music is a great way of getting extra motivation or inspiration. Mark Fenske, the co-author of *The Winner's Brain: 8 Strategies Great Minds Use to Achieve Success*, says that focusing on a favourite song combats de-motivating brain signals associated with fatigue or boredom. Much of music's power lies in its ability to elicit emotional reactions and enhance mood. This has been proven with neuro-imaging investigations showing how the sense of empowerment that can arise from a good set of lyrics, or the intensely positive memories associated with a favourite piece of music, actually stimulates motivation-related brain regions.[5] So, create a playlist of empowering upbeat songs that make you feel happy, hold good memories and make you feel energised. Mine include songs from Oasis, Take That and who can resist a bit of 'Moves Like Jagger' by Maroon 5? Play them when you're exercising to improve your motivation and endurance.

Body brushing will help the detoxification process by increasing the circulation to the skin and lymphatic drainage. This helps to encourage the body to release toxins. Body brushes are inexpensive to buy, so the good news is you can do this yourself at home. Use your brush on dry skin, starting at the ankles and working upwards in circular motions towards the heart as the lymphatic fluid flows towards the heart. The only exception is when you brush your back, which you can brush downwards if you wish. After the ankles, do the lower legs, thighs, stomach, back and arms. After this have a shower to wash away the impurities. Just five minutes a day is enough to see an improvement.

When you're going through a physical detox, it's also completely normal to feel more emotional than usual. By day four or five you will be feeling so much better – full of energy and vitality – so don't worry and instead focus on that fabulous end result.

The best bit about this plan is that you can eat as much as you want. There is no limit so you never have to feel hungry in week one, just as long as you are choosing healthy clean eating options. But as an added bonus, you will also lose some weight on this plan. The amount can vary from four to ten pounds in the first two weeks.

Need more motivation to carry on? Listen to what the gorgeous Elizabeth had to say after the cleanse:

Elizabeth's Experience

I got into bad habits over the last year including not eating my five a day and reaching for chocolate far too often! I also have IBS and dairy/wheat intolerances so my stomach is rarely completely peaceful. Firstly, the three-week cleanse has really helped me to incorporate so much more veg and fruit into my day that I'm blasting the five a day – it's more like eight! Next, I've reduced my cravings for bad sugar and found some lovely, natural alternatives. Without counting any calories I've also lost six pounds, which I'm delighted with. My stomach has been calmer – no bloating – and eating really 'clean' helps no end. Finally, the advice on supplements is brilliant, giving my body that extra support. Dr Sohère is a superb, down-to-earth advisor, whose advice you can really trust.

– Elizabeth Inniss, Birmingham, UK

WEEK TWO

The difference this week is that there are two liquid meals a day. I advise having a liquid breakfast and dinner, and having your big meal at lunchtime. This is so you have a long period for your digestive system to really rest and repair overnight. Having a big meal at lunchtime may seem tricky at work, but the key is preparation. Most workplaces have a microwave you can use to heat up a meal that you have pre-prepared the night before and brought to work in a container. There is no compelling evidence that microwaving food destroys nutrients, as long as you don't over-microwave your food (see page 107). If your workplace does not have a microwave or you don't like the idea of microwaving, you can make something that does not require heating up, like a large salad with couscous and cold meat. The amount of carbohydrates is also reduced this week.

The other change is the supplements that I recommend you take. Let's go through them now:

- **Probiotics** – to help have a healthy gut flora balance, improve digestive system function and help break down food.
- **Digestive enzymes** – to help your digestive system break down your food easily and absorb as much nutrition as possible from your meals.
- **Psyllium husk** – this is a natural fibre product that will encourage regular bowel function.
- **Omega-3 fatty acids** – essential for normal metabolism.
- **Multivitamin/wholefood supplement** – to ensure optimum nutrition.

So your programme will look like this:

Breakfast: juice or smoothie, psyllium husk , probiotics and digestive enzymes

Snack: hummus and vegetable sticks

Lunch: digestive enzymes/probiotics/omega-3 fish oils, protein and salad or vegetables with carbohydrates like brown rice, couscous or sweet potato

Snack: trail mix (see page 143) or nuts

> **Dinner**: wholefood supplement/multivitamin, probiotic and digestive enzymes. Soup, smoothie or protein and vegetables/salad (no carbohydrates at dinner) (see below)

If you are new to having liquid meals, you can start with one a day, for breakfast, and then by week three you can build up to the two liquid meals a day if you can manage it and it fits in with your lifestyle. If you want to you can have your liquid meals at breakfast and lunch, but you would have a deeper detox if you have them at breakfast and in the evening. If you really feel you cannot do this, just continue to eat clean.

Try to leave at least 12 hours between your evening liquid meal and morning liquid meal. This is to give your body ample time to rest and repair. Keep well hydrated with herbal teas or water, as often the body mistakes thirst for hunger. I don't want you to feel hungry so any time throughout the day when you do, and you have already drunk a glass of water, you can snack on fruit, trail mix (see page 143), vegetables and hummus, seeds or nuts. Just make sure it's a healthy option.

As I've said numerous times, I want this plan to fit in with your life, so if you have a dinner engagement you can't get out of, have your liquid or a light meal at lunchtime and choose a healthy option for dinner which is carbohydrate-free. This is fine to do now and again to fit in with your social life.

Only one week to go! Keep motivated by hearing how great Rachel felt after her three-week cleanse:

Rachel's Experience

Recently I developed bad habits with regards to eating. I would eat a lot of chocolate, takeaways and just junk in general! I hardly had any fruit or vegetables. I felt bloated, sluggish, tired and had no motivation.

Since doing this cleanse programme I have so much more energy, my concentration at work has increased and I feel better in myself. My clothes are also fitting better which is always good! The programme has also taught me good eating habits and a way to keep this up for the rest of my life. I'm never going back to my old ways!

– Rachel Freeman, Cardiff, UK

WEEK THREE

By now you will be feeling amazing and, hopefully, are completely used to the eating plan. It's now time to increase your exercise and also perform an 'emotional detox'.

EMOTIONAL DETOX

We have been concentrating on detoxing our bodies during the three-week cleanse, but just as it's unhelpful to eat well for one week and then go back into your bad habits for the next 51 weeks of the year, it's unhelpful to cleanse the body but not pay the same attention to your mind. Take some time to go through an emotional detox – aside from the benefits of making you think and act more positively, it will reinforce the positive changes you have made to your diet. By now your energy levels should have sky-rocketed, so it is a good time to focus on goals and resolve any issues, as physically and emotionally you should be feeling energised.

For an emotional detox I find it helpful to spend time reflecting honestly on what I want out of life, what I do well and what I haven't done so well. If something is on my mind, such as perhaps a conflict with a friend or loved one, I try to resolve it during this time so I can move on and it isn't draining my emotional energy. If there are things I want to achieve but haven't, I find this time useful to write a plan to achieve my goal within a realistic time frame. If I'm creating patterns and self-sabotaging certain things in my life I find it helpful to try and understand myself without judgement and see why I'm acting this way.

Set aside a couple of hours to do this, and also some time to reflect back on it a few days later. The more in tune you become with yourself, the greater the improvement you will see in your health, energy and quality of life.

JUICE CLEANSING

If you want to, do some juice cleansing during this week that will give your system a greater boost. Maybe you already eat healthily and want a deeper detox. This can last from three days to a week. There are lots of juice detox guides to help you, but as a general rule, having three to four juices a day, or home-made soups along-side taking psyllium husk to aid a colon cleanse, will have deep beneficial effects. This gives your digestive system a rest and having only vegetables and fruit will flood your system with nutrients.

During a juice detox you often get some withdrawal symptoms from caffeine and sugar, but after doing the week one programme you should not have any of those, and your appetite will have probably shrunk a little, making the juice detox a lot easier. Having a few 'all juice/liquid days' will really rest your digestive system and give your body a chance to re-energise.

Here's how Zairah felt after her first three-week cleanse:

Zairah's Experience

During the last year I had been overindulging and put on a bit of weight (I had gone up two dress sizes to be precise!). My diet consisted mainly of chocolate, biscuits, cake and take-aways. I hardly ever met the requirement for five fruit and veg a day. I constantly felt sluggish, over-tired and had no motivation to do anything.

After following this cleanse I have managed to cut out completely all the junk food and I am eating around at least 10 pieces of fruit and veg daily. I feel much more energised and have even started exercising daily. The best thing, however, was that I am a lot less bloated from all the processed food and as a result two inches have come off my waist. I feel embarrassed that I used to abuse my body with so much junk food. I feel so much better in myself and I definitely am never ever going back to my old ways, no way. I would much rather reach for an orange now than a bar of chocolate.

– Zairah Swallow, Cardiff, UK

PROGRESS CHART

As well as establishing a baseline for your fatigue (see pages 108–9), it's helpful to keep track of your daily progress. The aim is not to judge or be too hard on yourself, it's just to keep you on track so you see how you are doing. This is especially helpful if you don't have many On pages 124–7 supporting you who you can share your progress with. Below is a table that you can fill out, but if you do not want to write in this book, there is a link to a progress chart available to download on www.holistic-doctor.co.uk.

DAY 1	DAY 2	DAY 3
Got enough sleep?	Got enough sleep?	Got enough sleep?
Made healthy food choices?	Made healthy food choices?	Made healthy food choices?
Cheated?	Cheated?	Cheated?
Felt motivated?	Felt motivated?	Felt motivated?
Did 20 minutes of exercise?	Did 20 minutes of exercise?	Did 20 minutes of exercise?
Did 15 minutes of relaxation?	Did 15 minutes of relaxation?	Did 15 minutes of relaxation?
Used affirmations?	Used affirmations?	Used affirmations?
Resisted temptation?	Resisted temptation?	Resisted temptation?
Comments:	Comments:	Comments:

DAY 4	DAY 5	DAY 6
Got enough sleep?	Got enough sleep?	Got enough sleep?
Made healthy food choices?	Made healthy food choices?	Made healthy food choices?
Cheated?	Cheated?	Cheated?
Felt motivated?	Felt motivated?	Felt motivated?
Did 20 minutes of exercise?	Did 20 minutes of exercise?	Did 20 minutes of exercise?
Did 15 minutes of relaxation?	Did 15 minutes of relaxation?	Did 15 minutes of relaxation?
Used affirmations?	Used affirmations?	Used affirmations?
Resisted temptation?	Resisted temptation?	Resisted temptation?
Comments:	Comments:	Comments:

DAY 7	DAY 8	DAY 9
Having more restful sleep?	Having more restful sleep?	Having more restful sleep?
Made healthy food choices?	Made healthy food choices?	Made healthy food choices?
Cheated?	Cheated?	Cheated?
Felt motivated?	Felt motivated?	Felt motivated?
Did 20 minutes of exercise?	Did 20 minutes of exercise?	Did 20 minutes of exercise?
Did 15 minutes of relaxation?	Did 15 minutes of relaxation?	Did 15 minutes of relaxation?
Used affirmations?	Used affirmations?	Used affirmations?
Resisted temptation?	Resisted temptation?	Resisted temptation?
Felt more energised?	Felt more energised?	Felt more energised?
Had reduced cravings?	Had reduced cravings?	Had reduced cravings?
Comments:	Comments:	Comments:
DAY 10	DAY 11	DAY 12
Having more restful sleep?	Having more restful sleep?	Having more restful sleep?
Made healthy food choices?	Made healthy food choices?	Made healthy food choices?
Cheated?	Cheated?	Cheated?
Felt motivated?	Felt motivated?	Felt motivated?
Did 20 minutes of exercise?	Did 20 minutes of exercise?	Did 20 minutes of exercise?
Did 15 minutes of relaxation?	Did 15 minutes of relaxation?	Did 15 minutes of relaxation?
Used affirmations?	Used affirmations?	Used affirmations?
Resisted temptation?	Resisted temptation?	Resisted temptation?
Felt more energised?	Felt more energised?	Felt more energised?
Had reduced cravings?	Had reduced cravings?	Had reduced cravings?
Comments:	Comments:	Comments:

DAY 13	DAY 14	DAY 15
Felt great?	Resisted junk food?	Been lazy?
Having more restful sleep?	Having more restful sleep?	Having more restful sleep?
Made healthy food choices?	Made healthy food choices?	Made healthy food choices?
Cheated?	Cheated?	Cheated?
Felt motivated?	Felt motivated?	Felt motivated?
Did 20 minutes of exercise?	Did 20 minutes of exercise?	Did 20 minutes of exercise?
Did 15 minutes of relaxation?	Did 15 minutes of relaxation?	Did 15 minutes of relaxation?
Used affirmations?	Used affirmations?	Used affirmations?
Resisted temptation?	Resisted temptation?	Resisted temptation?
Felt more energised?	Felt more energised?	Felt more energised?
Had reduced cravings?	Had reduced cravings?	Had reduced cravings?
Comments:	Comments:	Comments:

DAY 16	DAY 17	DAY 18
Having more restful sleep?	Having more restful sleep?	Having more restful sleep?
Made healthy food choices?	Made healthy food choices?	Made healthy food choices?
Cheated?	Cheated?	Cheated?
Felt motivated?	Felt motivated?	Felt motivated?
Did 20 minutes of exercise?	Did 20 minutes of exercise?	Did 20 minutes of exercise?
Did 15 minutes of relaxation?	Did 15 minutes of relaxation?	Did 15 minutes of relaxation?
Used affirmations?	Used affirmations?	Used affirmations?
Resisted temptation?	Resisted temptation?	Resisted temptation?
Felt more energised?	Felt more energised?	Felt more energised?
Had reduced cravings?	Had reduced cravings?	Had reduced cravings?
Spent time doing an 'emotional detox'?	Made time to see good friends?	Taken time out to do something fun just for you?
Comments:	Comments:	Comments:

DAY 19	DAY 20	DAY 21
Having more restful sleep?	Having more restful sleep?	Having more restful sleep?
Made healthy food choices?	Made healthy food choices?	Made healthy food choices?
Cheated?	Cheated?	Cheated?
Felt motivated?	Felt motivated?	Felt motivated?
Did 20 minutes of exercise?	Did 20 minutes of exercise?	Did 20 minutes of exercise?
Did 15 minutes of relaxation?	Did 15 minutes of relaxation?	Did 15 minutes of relaxation?
Used affirmations?	Used affirmations?	Used affirmations?
Resisted temptation?	Resisted temptation?	Resisted temptation?
Felt more energised?	Felt more energised?	Felt more energised?
Had reduced cravings?	Had reduced cravings?	Had reduced cravings?
Made time to review your 'emotional detox'?	Made a plan to keep your energy up after finishing the 21-day programme?	Congratulate yourself on sticking with the programme. You are awesome!!!
Comments:	Comments:	Comments:

AFTER THE THREE-WEEK CLEANSE

The worst thing you can do after the cleanse is go on a massive binge of chocolate, cheese and bread. You will certainly feel the effects on your stomach – most people I know who have done that have spent a lot of time with cramps and in the toilet! You do not want to undo all your good work you have put in over the last three weeks.

My advice is to take things gradually. I would advise you to eat two 'clean' meals a day and then have small amounts of wheat and dairy if you want it for your third meal. It would also be good to have two completely 'clean' days in the week. This gives your body a chance to recover from any excesses.

If after following the three-week energy cleanse you don't feel 100 per cent well, there may be other imbalances that need correcting in the body. This normally requires further investigation and a more in-depth, personal consultation. If this is something you're worried about then please get in touch with a holistic health-care professional.

RECIPES

Here are some examples of recipes that are 'clean' for the eating plan. As you're able to eat as much 'good' food in this three-week cleanse, and as herbs and spices are a matter of taste, for some of these recipes, although I have stated amounts as guidance, it's important that you go with how your body feels: try to eat until you feel satisfied, but not stuffed.

BREAKFAST

Easy Almond Milk

1 handful of almonds, raw, unsalted
500 ml filtered or bottled water

Soak the almonds overnight. Drain and wash them. Then add to the water. Blend in a food processor, blender or use a hand blender until the mixture is completely smooth. Sieve the mixture to remove the small bits of almonds. Alternatively, you can strain the mixture with a cloth nut milk bag if you have one instead. The milk will keep for 24 to 48 hours. It must be refrigerated.

Protein Pancakes
Serves 1

> *2 mashed bananas*
> *2 eggs*
> *50 g vanilla protein powder*
> *1 tbsp coconut oil*
> *Optional ingredients: chopped blueberries, chopped strawberries*
> *Runny honey or peanut butter (organic, no additives) to serve*

Mix together the bananas, eggs and protein powder. Whisk or blend with a hand blender until smooth. If the mixture is a bit thick you can add almond milk or coconut water. Grease a frying pan with coconut oil and heat on a medium heat, and add the batter to the pan. Sprinkle the optional chopped fruit on top of the mixture. Cook on both sides for approximately one minute each. Serve with runny honey or peanut butter.

Quinoa and Fruit Cereal
Serves 1

> *150 g quinoa*
> *300 ml almond milk*
> *Chopped bananas, strawberries and blueberries*
> *Chopped mixed nuts*
> *Flax seeds and chia seeds*
> *Honey to taste*
> *Cinnamon to taste*

Make the quinoa as directed on the packet. Add the almond milk slowly, chopped fruit, nuts and seeds. Flavour with honey and cinnnamon according to your taste.

Healthy Granola

Makes up to 6 portions

175 g mixed nuts
450 g rolled oats
50 g sesame seeds
50 g sunflower seeds
50 g pumpkin seeds
Pinch of salt
25 ml olive oil
100 ml runny honey
85 g dried berries and cherries

Heat the oven to 190°C. Mix the nuts, oats, seeds and a pinch of salt in a large bowl. Add the oil and then the honey. Spoon onto a lined baking tray in a thin layer and bake for 20–25 minutes. When cooled break it up in to bite-size chunks. Add the dried fruit and store it in an airtight container. Serve with almond milk when ready to eat it.

Frittata

Serves 1

2 large eggs
Coarse salt and ground black pepper
1 tbsp extra-virgin olive oil
½ medium onion, finely chopped
1 handful of cherry tomatoes, halved
½ jalapeño pepper, finely chopped with seeds removed
A sprinkle of crumbled soft goat's cheese
¼ 400 g tin black beans, drained and rinsed

Whisk the eggs and season. Heat the oil in a frying pan and add the onion and tomatoes and cook until they have softened, approximately 5 minutes. Add in the eggs and the jalapeño pepper and cook until firm. Add the goat's cheese and then put the pan under the grill until the top begins to golden. Cook the beans separately as directed on the tin and then serve with the frittata.

Healthy Muesli
Makes up to 6 portions

> *450 g rolled oats (organic if possible)*
> *85 g mixed nuts*
> *100 g mixed seeds (pumpkin, sesame, sunflower)*
> *150 g dried fruit of your choice*
> *Soya, almond or rice milk or dairy-free yoghurt to serve*
> *Chopped fresh seasonal fruit, such as bananas, strawberries*
> *or blueberries to serve*

Mix all of the dry ingredients together and store in a large airtight container. To serve, spoon a portion into a bowl, pour over the milk or yoghurt and top with chopped fresh fruit.

JUICE AND SMOOTHIE RECIPES

Buying a juicer is one of the best investments I've ever made as I love juicing. I only have a basic juicer but it's made a huge difference to my nutrition. There has been some bad press about juices and smoothies as they're full of sugar, but I'd like to point out these studies have been done on shop-bought smoothies and juices that have been pasteurised and have lost their nutritional content, *not* freshly made juices. Pasteurised juices have been heated up and all the nutrients have been killed, so in essence you are drinking a glass of sugar. In some parts of the country you can buy fresh juice or cold-pressed juice, or order it from companies online. Sometimes I make my juices in advance and freeze them. There's a lot of conflicting information about whether this depletes the nutritional value, and of course the best option is to make your juice fresh and drink it immediately, but if this isn't possible then I think that if you have to make your juices in advance or freeze them, this is still a better option than eating something unhealthy. It's about making the best decision with the time and resources you have.

Below are some examples of juices you can try at home, although there are lots of other great resources for juice recipes out there. In my opinion, there are few better ways to start your day than with a Green Smoothie!

Piña Colada
Serves 1

> *1 30 g scoop of vanilla-flavoured protein powder or plain whey or hemp protein powder with 3 drops of natural vanilla essence (unsweetened) added*
> *½ medium pineapple, fresh*
> *250 ml coconut milk (unsweetened)*

Peel the pineapple and cut into small chunks. Blend the ingredients together in a blender. Add water or coconut water if too thick. Add ice if you prefer it chilled.

Berry Delight
Serves 1

> *1 30 g scoop of vanilla-flavoured protein powder*
> *250 ml coconut or almond milk*
> *2 handfuls of strawberries/raspberries/blueberries (frozen or fresh)*

Wash the berries if fresh and blend the ingredients together in a blender until smooth.

Banana Blast
Serves 1

> *1 30 g scoop of vanilla-flavoured protein powder*
> *1 medium banana, peeled*
> *300 ml almond milk*
> *1 tbsp runny or manuka honey*

Blend the ingredients together in a blender until smooth.

Tony's Breakfast Smoothie

Inspired by my good friend Tony Munoz, and my absolute favourite.
Serves 1

1 30 g scoop of vanilla or chocolate-flavoured protein powder
300 ml dairy-free milk – almond, soy or rice
75 g rolled oats (organic if possible)
1 tbsp organic peanut butter with no additives
1 medium banana peeled
100 ml coconut water

Blend the ingredients together in a blender or use a hand blender until smooth.

Immune Blast

Serves 1

1 medium apple, unpeeled
3 medium carrots, unpeeled
2 medium oranges, peeled
6-mm piece ginger root, unpeeled, or to taste
½ lemon (unwaxed if you want to juice in the rind,
 otherwise peel)

Juice the ingredients and enjoy.

Green Smoothie

Serves 1

1 medium apple, unpeeled
4 slices fresh pineapple, peeled
2 large handfuls of spinach or kale
½ avocado, peeled and stone removed
⅓ cucumber, unpeeled
5-cm piece broccoli stem
2 sticks of celery

Wash the apple, spinach or kale, cucumber, broccoli and celery.
Blend the ingredients together in a blender until smooth.

Mango Delight
Serves 1

¼ medium mango, peeled and stone removed
1 medium apple, unpeeled
2 large handfuls of spinach
2 sprigs of fresh mint
100 ml coconut water

Wash the apple, spinach and mint. Blend the ingredients together in a blender until smooth. Add a teaspoon of wheat grass or spirulina powder for an added energy and nutrient boost.

Beetroot Beauty
Serves 1

1 small beetroot – raw, unpeeled
2 large handfuls of spinach
2 medium apples, unpeeled
2 cm root ginger, unpeeled

Wash all ingredients and pass them through juicer whole.

Sweet Treat
This isn't a good one to have every day, but as a treat from time to time it's fine. It's also a great hangover cure!
Serves 1

1 kiwi, peeled
2 medium apples, unpeeled
5 slices of fresh pineapple, peeled
2 tbsp of dairy-free yoghurt
1 large handful of blueberries

Wash the apples and blueberries. Put the apples, kiwi and pineapple through a juicer. Transfer the juice to a blender, add the yoghurt and blueberries, blend until smooth.

SALADS AND HOT DISHES FOR LUNCH AND DINNER

Vegetable and Bean Chilli
Serves 4

> *1 large onion, chopped*
> *1 clove of garlic, chopped*
> *1 chilli, finely chopped*
> *1 tsp paprika*
> *1 tsp chilli powder*
> *½ tsp turmeric*
> *400 g tin chopped tomatoes*
> *Approximately 200 g of roughly chopped vegetables, these*
>   *can include: mushrooms, carrots, broccoli, leeks,*
>   *aubergine, peas, sweetcorn*
> *400 g tin mixed pulses (kidney beans, butter beans, chick*
>   *peas)*
> *1 tsp dried rosemary*
> *1 handful spinach*
> *Brown rice or couscous to serve*

Quick-fry onion, garlic, chilli, paprika, chilli powder and turmeric in 1 tbsp of olive oil or coconut oil on a medium heat until ingredients have softened. Add tomatoes and vegetables. Add mixed pulses and rosemary. Add 300ml water and leave to simmer for 30 minutes until reduced.

Add spinach at end while on the heat and cook for 1–2 minutes.

Serve with brown rice or couscous.

Stir-fry
Serves 2

1 tbsp coconut oil
1 clove of garlic, chopped
2.5 cm piece ginger
1 chilli, finely chopped
1 large onion, finely chopped
1 tbsp coconut oil
300 g finely sliced vegetables, these can include: mushrooms,
*   peppers, water chestnuts, broccoli, carrot, baby corn,*
*   mangetout, pak choi*
Lean protein such as chicken, turkey, prawns or tofu –
*   approximately 200 g*
1–2 tbsp soy sauce
1 large handful of cashew nuts
Sesame oil to serve
Brown rice or rice noodles to serve

Quick-fry garlic, ginger, onion and chilli in the coconut oil. Add vegetables and protein and stir-fry until cooked, add soy sauce. Toast some cashews in a separate pan and add to the stir-fry. Drizzle with sesame oil before serving.

Serve with brown rice or rice noodles.

Easy Tomato Sauce
Serves 2

1 tbsp coconut oil
2 cloves of garlic, chopped
1 small chilli, finely chopped
1 medium onion, finely chopped
1 handful of chopped anchovies and olives
Optional protein such as chicken, prawns, tuna, turkey
Approximately 300 g of diced mushrooms, broccoli, red and
*   yellow peppers, sun-dried tomatoes, aubergine*

400 g tin chopped tomatoes
A pinch of dried oregano
1 handful of spinach
1 handful of fresh basil
Brown rice or couscous to serve

Quick-fry garlic, chilli and onion with some coconut oil. Add the chopped anchovies and olives and stir-fry for 1 minute. Add in protein if you have opted for it and then all the vegetables, tomatoes and oregano. Leave to simmer for 30 minutes.

Add handful of spinach and basil towards the end of cooking. Serve with brown rice or couscous.

Quinoa Salad
Serves 1

Any vegetable that is good to grill or roast, suggestions
*   include handful of mushrooms, 1 pepper, 1 onion,*
*   1 large aubergine, 1 courgette*
1 clove crushed garlic
Lemon juice
Wholegrain mustard
Olive oil/Hemp oil/flax oil.
200 g quinoa
1 handful of chopped olives
1 handful of sundried tomatoes
50 g cherry tomatoes
50 g halved baby corn
1 handful of raisins
Diced feta cheese (make sure it is made from goat's milk
*   not cow's milk)*
Green leafy salad to serve
Lean chicken or fish, optional to serve

Grill or dry-roast the vegetables. Cook the quinoa according to packet instructions. In a separate bowl mix crushed garlic, lemon juice, wholegrain mustard and oil. Stir the vegetables, sundried tomatoes, olives, cherry tomatoes, baby corn, raisins and feta cheese into the quinoa and add the garlic dressing.

Serve with a green leafy salad and, if you wish, some lean cooked chicken or fish.

Prawn Salad
Serves 1

> *1 small lettuce*
> *1 ripe avocado, peeled with stone removed*
> *2 medium oranges, peeled*
> *140 g cooked king prawns*
> *1 small red onion, finely chopped*
> *Small bunch coriander, leaves picked*
> *Juice of ½ lime*

Chop the lettuce roughly. Slice the avocado and oranges and arrange over the lettuce. Add the prawns, finely chopped red onion and coriander. Squeeze the lime juice over the salad and mix.

Salmon and Brown Rice Salad
Serves 2

> *200 g brown rice*
> *200 g frozen peas, defrosted*
> *2 salmon fillets, approx 250 g*
> *1 cucumber, diced*
> *Small bunch spring onions, sliced*
> *Small bunch coriander, roughly chopped*
> *1 red chilli, diced with seeds removed*
> *Zest and juice of 1 lime*
> *4 tsp light soy sauce*

Cook the rice according to the instructions on the pack and 5 minutes before it is cooked add the frozen peas. Drain the rice and put it in a dish. Grill the salmon until it is cooked, approximately 15–20 minutes. Remove the skin and flake the salmon and add it to the rice. Take the cucumber, spring onion, coriander, chilli and mix with the lime zest and juice and soy sauce. Pour this over the rice and salmon, mix thoroughly and serve.

Spicy Chicken and Broccoli
Serves 1

> *1 broccoli head, cut into florets*
> *Salt and freshly ground black pepper*
> *1 clove of garlic, finely chopped*
> *2 shallots, finely sliced*
> *½ red chilli, sliced with seeds removed*
> *1 tbsp olive oil*
> *1 roasted chicken breast, sliced*
> *1 tbsp soy sauce*
> *1 handful pitted black olives*

Steam the broccoli and season it.

Fry the garlic, shallots and chilli in the olive oil until softened. Mix with the olives, broccoli and sliced chicken. Add the soy sauce and season to taste. This can be eaten warm or cold.

Easy Salad Dressing
Makes up to 6 servings

> *50 ml balsamic vinegar*
> *200 ml olive oil/flax oil/hemp oil*
> *2 tsp lemon juice*
> *1–2 cloves of crushed garlic*
> *Freshly ground black pepper to taste*
> *2 tsp of dried oregano*

Mix all ingredients together and drizzle on salads and vegetables. This can be made and kept to use as needed over the cleanse period. Store in a glass jar or container and keep for a maximum of 2 weeks.

Fish or Chicken Bake

Serves 2

This is a complete meal as it has a balance of carbohydrates, proteins and vegetables all included in it.

1 red pepper
1 small red onion, peeled
2 medium carrots, peeled
1 small courgette
1 small potato, peeled
3 tbsp olive or coconut oil
3 tsp mixed dried herbs
3 garlic cloves, peeled and crushed
2 fillets of salmon or white fish or 2 chicken breasts
1 tsp chilli powder
Salt and freshly ground black pepper to taste

Preheat the oven to 180°C. Roughly chop the vegetables and place in an oven tray, coat with olive or coconut oil, half of the mixed herbs and half of the crushed garlic, roast for 30–45 minutes, checking and turning regularly.

In a separate baking tray, coat the chicken or fish in a mix of chilli powder, the remaining garlic and mixed herbs and salt and pepper to taste. Bake in the oven for approximately 20-30 minutes for fish, or 25–35 minutes for chicken. Serve the chicken of fish with the roasted vegetables.

SOUPS

Slow-roasted Cherry Tomato and Pepper Soup

Serves 2

4 cloves of garlic
2 small punnets of ripe cherry tomatoes
1 red onion

2 red peppers, roughly chopped
1 tbsp olive oil
500 ml vegetable stock
1 tbsp dried mixed herbs or to taste
Salt and freshly ground black pepper to taste

Preheat the oven to 190°C. Place the garlic, tomatoes, onion and peppers in a roasting tin. Drizzle with the olive oil and roast for approximately 30–45 minutes. Boil the stock and then add the vegetables. Put into a blender and blend with the dried herbs. Add salt and pepper to taste.

Leek and Sweet Potato Soup

2 sweet potatoes, peeled
2 leeks
600 ml chicken or vegetable stock
Salt and freshly ground pepper to taste
Dried mixed herbs to taste

Roughly cut the potatoes and leeks. Boil the potatoes and leeks in the stock until the potatoes are soft. Blend in a blender or with a hand blender. Add salt and pepper and mixed herbs to taste.

You can substitute the leeks with celery if you wish.

Sweet Potato and Vegetable Soup

3 sweet potatoes, peeled and chopped
3 carrots, peeled and chopped
3 sticks of celery, finally chopped
1 small tin sweetcorn
Mixed dried herbs
Salt and freshly ground black pepper
600 ml vegetable stock

Season the vegetables with herbs, pepper and a pinch of salt and boil in the stock until soft.

Blend in a blender or with a hand blender and season to taste.

Chicken and Mushroom Soup

> *Small punnet of mushrooms, washed and chopped*
> *1 onion finely chopped*
> *1 medium chicken breast*
> *500 ml boiling vegetable or chicken stock*
> *Mixed dried herbs*
> *Salt and freshly ground black pepper*

Pan-fry the mushrooms and onion, for 10 minutes while roasting the chicken in the oven at 180°C for 20–25 minutes.

Cut the chicken into very small pieces and then blend the chicken and vegetables all together with the stock. Season with herbs and salt and pepper to taste.

SWEETS AND SNACKS

Who says you can't have a delicious treat when on a cleanse? Below are some healthy suggestions when you feel like you need a dessert or snack. Raw cacao or cocoa powder is fine to consume when it hasn't been processed.

Chocolate Mousse
Serves 4

> *4 fresh pitted dates*
> *2 ripe avocados, skin and stones removed*
> *1 medium ripe banana, chopped*
> *1 tsp natural vanilla extract*
> *100 g raw cacao powder or cocoa powder*
> *Pinch of sea salt and cinnamon to enhance flavour*

Combine all the ingredients in a blender. Blend until smooth and creamy. Add a splash of water or coconut water to make a lighter mousse. Spoon into a bowl and allow to set in the fridge.

Brownies
4–6 portions

120 g pecans or walnuts
150 g fresh pitted dates
5 tbsp raw cacao (cocoa) powder
4 tbsp shredded unsweetened coconut
2 tbsp runny honey or agave nectar
¼ tsp sea salt

Blend the nuts in a food processor until crumbly. Add the dates and blend again until soft. Add the remaining ingredients and blend until you have an even brown mixture that should not be too liquidy. Spoon the mixture into a baking tray and pat down. Refrigerate for 2–4 hours. Then cut the brownies into squares. These can be stored in an airtight container in the fridge for about a week.

Flapjacks
12 portions

2 tbsp olive oil, plus a little extra for greasing
2 tbsp smooth organic peanut butter
3 tbsp runny honey or agave syrup
2 ripe bananas, mashed
1 apple, peeled, cored and grated
150 g rolled oats (organic if possible)
100 ml hot water
50 g chopped nuts
100 g raisins or cranberries
85 g mixed seeds (pumpkin, sunflower and sesame)
25 g dessicated coconut

Preheat oven to 160°C. Grease and line a 20cm square tin with baking paper. Heat the oil, peanut butter and honey or agave syrup in a small pan until melted. Add the mashed banana, apple and

100ml hot water, and mix. Add the oats, dried fruit, dessicated coconut and the seeds and stir until everything is mixed. Tip into the tin. Bake for 45 minutes or until golden. Leave to cool and then cut into pieces. These can be stored in an airtight container in the fridge for about a week.

Trail Mix

This is really popular in the USA. You can keep it on your desk at work or in your bag so you always have something healthy to snack on. You need a mixture of unsalted nuts, dried fruits such as berries, raisins, apples and banana pieces and mixed seeds.

If you are looking for a natural way to reboot your energy, kick-start a healthier way of life or drop a few pounds, this three-week energy cleanse could be the answer you've been searching for.

Remember, preparation is the key, and be kind to yourself, as if you are doing this while working a full-time job or looking after small children you may slip up. This doesn't mean you have to give up! This is about you taking control of your energy and health and it is not a disaster if you have one bad day. You will reap the rewards by making these changes for a short time and giving your body a chance to repair and recuperate. Even better, if you can encourage a few friends or family members to do this with you, you will be able to support and encourage each other in your quest for better energy and wellness. If the full three weeks seems daunting, why not try one week and see how you get on? I am so sure you will feel so much better that you will want to keep going for the next two weeks. Give it a go and take control of your wellness and energy!

CHAPTER 10
SLEEP WELL

As well as eating well, sleep is so important to feel rested, energised, and to help the body to recover and do essential repair work.

> **Did you know...**
> - Poor sleep can cause heart problems and depression?
> - Your mobile phone might be stopping you from sleeping?
> - Lack of sleep might be making you fat?
> - Getting good sleep can keep you looking younger for longer?

Restful sleep is vital to allow the body to regenerate, but many of us struggle with getting it. The side effects of poor sleep habits include memory loss, confusion, high blood pressure, obesity, cardiovascular disease and depression.

Virtually every system in your body is affected by the amount and quality of sleep you get. The benefits of good sleep include: weight loss, as sleep regulates the amount you eat and how your metabolism works; natural immunity to fight off infections; better coping mechanisms; increased ability to learn new things, including improving your memory, creativity and insightfulness.

Sleep governs our 'circadian rhythm', which means our body's natural internal clock. Certain hormones in our body are produced at specific times of the day and night, either to give us energy in the day, or to help repair the body overnight. Irregular sleep leads to these hormones not being secreted in their correct amounts, and can make us feel tired in the day, and reduce the regeneration of the body's cells at night.

SIGNS YOU ARE NOT GETTING ENOUGH SLEEP

1. WAKING UP FEELING TIRED

This may seem obvious, but if you wake up every day and still feel tired whether you have had five hours' sleep or nine, you are probably sleep deprived. The body hasn't had enough time to regenerate and rest and the constant changes in sleep patterns is not allowing time to recover.

2. RELYING ON SUGAR AND CAFFEINE TO KEEP GOING

If you have strong sugar and caffeine cravings it could be due to the fact you are not getting enough sleep. The stimulating effects of sugar and caffeine is your body responding to lack of sleep to keep going.

3. LAPSES IN CONCENTRATION AND FOCUS

When you are tired it can be hard to concentrate and you may find yourself making 'silly' mistakes at work. Researchers discovered that after you've gone a night without sleep, you're essentially operating on the same level as someone who's intoxicated by alcohol. Sleep deprivation leads to slower reaction times. Studies show it affects speed before it affects accuracy (be it physical or mental). Lack of sleep has also been shown to lead to poorer decision making and taking unnecessary risks.

4. YOU KEEP GETTING COLDS

Poor immunity can be caused by a lack of sleep. A study found that people who sleep less than seven hours a night are almost three times as likely to catch a cold than those who sleep more than seven hours. Your white blood cells which fight infection become less in number, and those remaining become less effective.[1]

5. YOU ARE HUNGRY ALL THE TIME

Sleep-deprived people have a higher than normal level of ghrelin, the hunger hormone. This increases snacking and also the craving for carbohydrate foods.

6. YOU ARE PUTTING ON WEIGHT

Because of the increased levels of ghrelin, the hunger hormone, those who are sleep deprived are at greater risk of obesity.

7. YOU FEEL YOU ARE CLUMSIER THAN USUAL

Reflexes are dulled when tired, so balance and depth perception can be a little wonky. As well as having trouble focusing, reaction time can be slowed, meaning you can't quite catch the egg carton before it hits the floor.

8. YOU FEEL DOWN IN THE DUMPS

If you find yourself tearful and weepy and low in mood it could be due to lack of sleep, as it can affect hormones and also the brain's ability to deal with emotional experiences.

9. YOU'VE LOST YOUR SEX DRIVE

Tiredness can affect your sex drive due to low energy and also an increase in cortisol, the stress hormone.

10. WORSENING MEDICAL PROBLEMS

People with conditions such as diabetes and high blood pressure can experience no improvement in their condition due to lack of sleep. Diabetics who are sleep deprived become less sensitive to insulin.

MEDICAL CAUSES OF POOR SLEEP

Of course, there may be medical reasons for why you can't sleep, for instance, if you are in physical pain or suffer from depression. If this is the case, it is certainly worth visiting your doctor to see if anything can be done to help.

Another cause of poor and restless sleep is a condition called sleep apnoea. The symptoms of sleep apnoea include snoring, waking up with a headache, feeling moody, congested and extremely tired during the day. More details can be found in chapter 2 (see pages 23–4).

Beauty benefits

Getting good sleep isn't just going to get rid of the bags under your eyes. While you sleep, your skin is not being exposed to damaging free radicals, UV light or environmental factors that can cause harm. As the body doesn't have to protect the skin overnight, it can use energy to repair any damage, such as fine lines and wrinkles. Therefore any products you use to hydrate or repair the skin will be extra effective overnight. Moreover, a study published in the *British Medical Journal* in 2010 showed that women who had eight hours' sleep a night were perceived as better-looking than when they had five hours' sleep. So we really do need our beauty sleep![2]

SUPPLEMENTS TO AID SLEEP

It's always worthwhile trying other methods – such as turning off your computer an hour before bed and spending some time relaxing (there are more tips on pages 151–4), such as those listed further along in this chapter – but when you feel like you need some extra help to drop off, or need to reset your sleep patterns, supplements can help.

- **Melatonin** is a natural hormone made by the body that helps regulate the sleep-waking cycle. It helps people fall asleep and also enhances the quality of sleep. Melatonin is useful to take to combat jet lag, and is safe to take for short-term use to regulate the sleep cycle. In the UK it is difficult to get this prescribed on the NHS. A dose between 3–9 milligrams a night is recommended.
- **Valerian** is a root that has been used as a sedative and to reduce anxiety for thousands of years. It is readily available in health-food shops and many people feel it improves their sleep. It is not a good idea to take it with alcohol or other sleep medications. It becomes more effective with time so it could be a few days before you start feeling the benefits. Start with a dose of 400mg a night but it can be increased as necessary.
- **5-HTP** helps make serotonin and can induce sleep. It also aids mood and decreases appetite. It is not recommended for those on antidepressants.
- **Magnesium** is essential for a good night's sleep and also for helping normal muscle and nerve function, keeping the heart rate steady, regulating blood sugars, maintaining a healthy blood pressure, keeping bones strong and maintaining a healthy immune system. Low levels of magnesium in the body can cause stress and nervousness in a person, and can reduce sleep quality and cause a person to wake up in the night.

- **Theanine** is an amino acid that is found in green tea and can be taken in supplement form. It can trigger the release of GABA (gamma-aminobutyric acid). GABA aids relaxation and reduces anxiety, but is difficult to absorb from a supplement. A dose of 600mg of theanine each day can be taken safely without supervision by a health-care professional.

Sleeping pills?

People frequently consult their doctor for sleeping pills. Sometimes they are prescribed short term for a few days to help 'reset' one's sleeping pattern or during a time of extreme emotional distress. Most doctors are reluctant to prescribe them long term for very good reasons:

- Sleeping tablets can be addictive, both physically and psychologically
- They can leave you feeling drowsy or 'hungover' the next day
- They may help you get to sleep, but they don't encourage the deep sleep needed for regeneration of the body and hormone regulation previously mentioned
- There has even been some recent evidence that taking sleeping tablets long term can cause premature death[3]

I often use the analogy that you're just putting a plaster over a cut that doesn't heal. Essentially, you're not getting to the root of why you cannot sleep.

TOP TIPS TO IMPROVE YOUR SLEEP TONIGHT

Here are some healthy habits to get into to improve your chances of getting a good night's sleep.

- Turn off your TV/computer/smartphone an hour before you go to bed. Electrical appliances stimulate the brain and won't aid sleep. Reading is also too stimulating. Who hasn't decided to read just one last chapter of their book before bed and found themselves still engrossed at 2 a.m.?
- Try and get into a bedtime routine, like when you were a child. Take at least 30 minutes to wind down. You can listen to relaxing music and use the time to take stock of your day. Don't use the time to do chores or watch TV dramas.
- Take a hot bath. A night's sleep is normally preceded by a drop in body temperature. When you have a comfortably hot bath, artificially raising your body temperature, when you go back into your cooler bedroom it helps the body be more receptive to adjusting its body temperature.
- Warm skimmed milk (organic if possible) aids sleep, as do bananas. Both release natural chemicals to relax the body and help you fall asleep due to their calcium content. They also both contain tryptophan, which can be converted into serotonin by the body which can help you to feel sleepy. Skimmed milk is preferable as full-fat milk can put a burden on our digestive system and keep us awake at night. Nuts such as Brazil nuts and walnuts also induce sleep due to being packed with protein, potassium and selenium and can help the body make melatonin, the natural sleep hormone. Kale and spinach are also rich in calcium and can help the body to produce tryptophan and melatonin. Chickpeas (the main ingredient of hummus), shrimp and lobster are rich sources of tryptophan.

- Almonds are rich in magnesium, which is essential for a good night's sleep. If magnesium levels are low, it is hard to stay asleep. You can also take a magnesium supplement to help you get to sleep.

- Can a salad for dinner help you sleep? Yes. Lettuce contains lactucarium, which has sedative properties and relaxes the brain. You can make a lettuce tea by simmering a few lettuce leaves in hot water for 10–15 minutes and sip before going to bed.

- Your body needs vitamin B6 to help make melatonin and serotonin. Foods rich in B6 are fish like tuna, halibut and salmon, as well as raw garlic and pistachio nuts.

- Certain foods that can raise the glycaemic index can induce sleep. This is because after eating them you have a natural spike in your blood sugar and insulin levels, and after this spike you can feel tired. Normally you want steady blood sugars in the day to avoid mood and energy swings, but if you are looking to get rest, this could help. Foods like white rice can help this process.

- Chamomile tea really can help sleep. It contains glycine, which relaxes nerves and muscles and can act as a mild sedative and also help reduce any anxiety. A little bit of honey in your chamomile tea can help too as it raises insulin and tryptophan.

- Carbohydrates at night can help induce sleep, such as rice, sweet potatoes, wholewheat pasta.

- Passion-flower tea has been found to promote good sleep.

- Some people find acupuncture, Ayurvedic medicine or traditional Chinese medicine helps them restore a good sleep cycle. Acupuncture is thought to increase melatonin in the body. Traditional Chinese medicine believes that insomnia stems from weak kidney energy and works to restore this. Ayurvedic medicine believes insomnia is often related to a vata imbalance. Vata regulates breathing and circulation. One type of treatment involves using oils on the head and the feet.

It is best to see specialist practitioners in these fields if you need further guidance.

- Avoid caffeine, sugar and alcohol. Caffeine and sugar shouldn't be consumed late in the day as they have been proven to cause restless sleep. Consider making 2 p.m. your cut-off time for caffeinated drinks if you're having trouble sleeping. Some people believe alcohol helps them sleep, but it actually leads to a less regenerative slumber, so the body doesn't rest well and you feel tired the next day. This is because alcohol disturbs chemicals in the brain that help with the deeper patterns of sleep. What actually happens is that brain waves increase from small ones in Stage One to deep slow waves in Stage Four. Stage Four is the deepest level of sleep that makes us refreshed the next day. But as alcohol starts to wear off during the night, we experience more Stage Five sleep – known as Rapid Eye Movement (REM) – than Stage Four. During this period, there is a high level of brain activity. Although this stage is associated with dreaming, it is a lighter type of sleep which is not as refreshing as Stage Four – and can affect our mental performance and mood during the next day.

- A few drops of lavender oil on the pillow are relaxing, but more than that is stimulating so use with caution.

- If your mattress and pillows are worn out or if your bed is more than 10 years old, invest in new ones as soon as possible. Studies have shown that buying a new bed can be more effective than sleeping pills and can improve a night's sleep by 42 minutes.

- Psychologically, if you spend all night wide awake and tossing and turning in your bed, you can think negatively of your bed. So for 20 minutes try to get to sleep and if you can't, get up, and read something relaxing or do something sedentary until you can. In the same way, the bedroom should only be used for bedroom activities, and not for watching TV or eating, to create a more relaxed sleep-inducing atmosphere.

- If you have a digital clock in your room, I'm afraid you're going to have to turn it off, as well as your phone. Both release electromagnetic waves into the room that can interrupt sleep. Consider turning your Wi-Fi off too for the same reason.
- Along a similar vein, make sure your room is as dark and quiet as possible. Invest in an eye mask and earplugs if needed.
- Try to sleep the same amount of hours every night and go to bed and wake up at roughly the same time, even at weekends, if possible. This allows your body to know when to secrete your hormones and make repairs, and doesn't confuse it with too many late nights. By going to bed at 11 p.m. one night and 3 a.m. the next, it can induce a mini 'jet lag' where our body becomes out of sync. This means we cannot get into Stage Four deep sleep, and this can affect our energy, mental performance and judgement the next day. It may sound boring, but getting into a routine with your sleep is a great way to regain your vitality.

ACTION PLAN

I know from my own experiences how frustrating it can be when you can't sleep and you wake up feeling tired before having to face a busy day. It's really important to get good sleep not only to feel energised, but to allow the body to carry out important reparative processes to keep you in good health. The tips above will help you improve your sleep hygiene. There are a lot of points above, so why don't you start by choosing three and implement them this week to try and improve your sleep. If they are not as effective as you would wish, then try some different ones the week after until you find the ones that work best for you.

CHAPTER 11
LESS STRESS, MORE ENERGY

Let's start with a clear definition of stress. There are many different types and explanations but the most common is that it is: *a condition or feeling experienced when a person perceives that demands exceed the personal and social resources he or she is able to mobilise.*[1] Another definition, even more relevant for our purposes, is that stress is not having *enough energy* to meet the demands of life.

We have so many opportunities and choices in our modern lives, yet, ironically, this brings its own stresses. We are now all too busy to do simple, important things such as going for walks in nature and cooking a healthy meal from scratch. We're switched on all the time and accessible 24 hours a day via our mobiles and the Internet. The result? Consistently high stress levels and the inability to relax properly.

Stress has a massive impact on our physical and mental health – it even affects our genes. In the past we thought our genes were fixed and there was nothing we could do to influence them. Now we know change is absolutely possible and it all begins with our telomeres; the bits on the end of our chromosomes that keep them intact, like the plastic caps that hold the ends of shoelaces together.

As cells divide and replicate, telomeres eventually shorten. When they become too short, the cells die and our lives become shorter as a result. Lots of different factors affect the shortening of the telomeres and Nobel Prize-winning research has shown that stress affects this shortening as much as smoking does. So, *stress is as bad for your health as smoking*![2] The great news is you can rejuvenate your cells by making simple health and lifestyle changes which I'll explain shortly.

Cultivating a peaceful mind is important for our health and energy levels, yet it's one of the last things we address (if we ever try). Statistics show one in four people develop depressive symptoms in their life. The rates are even higher for those with chronic disease: 8 per cent have major depression and up to 36 per cent have depressive symptoms.[3]

Psychoneuroimmunology (PNI) is the study of the interaction between psychological processes and the nervous and immune systems within the human body. PNI has shown how stress can negatively cause heart attacks, worsen outcomes in cancer and how depression can affect the progression of diseases such as HIV by directly affecting immune cells.

But the solution isn't just about finding ways to relax and manage stress. It's also about feeling happy and fulfilled, having a purpose in life and surrounding ourselves with people who make us feel good and give us support. These are the things that make life worth living.

It takes a lot of energy to process and recall our thoughts and create new ideas. Have you ever noticed that when you are with someone who is very negative you leave feeling absolutely drained after? Or how a walk in fresh air when the sun is shining makes you feel full of vitality even if you had been feeling sluggish before? Have you ever noticed when you're really tired that you can somehow become rejuvenated after spending a great evening with friends, laughing and having fun? I may feel tired, but if I'm having a good day at work seeing patients who are making great changes in their lives, or perhaps lecturing a group of people who are really interested in what I'm saying, I then feel energised and fresh – no matter how much sleep I've had the night before. This isn't the sort of energy that comes from the calories in our food, it is the energy that connects us to our internal source of energy and to our true self.

Below are my top tips on how to manage stress, feel energised, get happier and find fulfilment. Some may resonate more with you than others. That's okay. We're all individuals so take the time to consider those that work best for you.

APPRECIATION

We live in hectic times and, as we're always striving for more, we tend to miss out on what we already have. We're bombarded by messages in the media that tell us we should be slimmer, prettier, have a bigger house, a faster car or a better boyfriend so it's easy to feel unfulfilled. I know I do on occasion. Beyoncé Knowles and I are the same age and I went through a phase of looking at her and feeling highly unsatisfied with my life and thinking I was completely inadequate! Worries and fears drain our energy and stop us from using our precious resources for more important things. The solution is gratitude. Being grateful for what you have is a great antidote to stress and dissatisfaction, and serves as a reminder of the good things in our lives. So, I firmly recommend you keep a gratitude journal.

Every morning write down three things you are grateful for and do the same before bed as you reflect on the day. It can be as simple as enjoying a cup of tea with a good friend or feeling happy the sun has been shining. Remembering the positive aspects of yourself and your life will have a positive effect on your mental well-being and mood. You don't have to write these things down, but the reason I find recording my gratitude useful myself is because when I have a 'down' day, it's lovely to read over all the memories, events and happy occasions that have happened over time and remember things aren't that bad really, even if I don't have Beyoncé's life!

CREATIVE VISUALISATION

Scientific research and the study of PNI have shown that visualising can make a positive difference to our health. Amazingly, cancer sufferers who spend time visualising their cancer cells being destroyed have better results in beating the disease than those who don't.[4] Were you ever told not to daydream as a child? This is the proof the naysayers were wrong!

Certain situations can make us feel helpless and this in turn causes stress. Accepting and letting go of things we can't control is a first step, but it can also be helpful to spend time visualising – or imagining – the life we want.

Simply sit comfortably, close your eyes and imagine the life you want and the person you want to be. Engage your senses, first your sight by seeing the colours in your mind's eye, then your hearing by imagining you can hear the relevant sounds. If you want to use this to increase your energy, see the best 'you' you can – full of energy, looking fantastic, being able to do all the things you want to in a day. Allow the feelings of joy, lightness and energy to fill you to make it real. This only takes five minutes a day and can have huge benefits on your health and mood.

BREATHE

You may be wondering why something as natural as breathing gets its own section, but there's a correct way to breathe for maximum energy and stress relief. We often breathe unconsciously, but it's important to become aware of how we breathe as we often develop poor habits.

Studies have shown that dysfunctional breathing affects the heart rate variability and this can worsen asthma, stress, blood pressure and cardiorespiratory problems.[5] Breathing in a regular rhythm has an effect on the heart and health in general. The best way to breathe is to make the out-breath slightly longer than the in-breath. Any pattern of this is good, but the ideal is four seconds in, and seven seconds out. Practise this for five minutes a day, before bed or whenever you're relaxing.

It's also beneficial to use your stomach while breathing, known as abdominal breathing. A technique often practised by yoga followers is to push the stomach out when breathing in, inflating it like a balloon, and then to flatten it, deflating the balloon, on the out-breath. It may feel a bit odd at first but with a little practice this will soon become routine.

A breathing technique to reduce stress is to breathe in eight times and then take one long breath out. This can be repeated for about five minutes to try and calm the mind.

The breath of fire is one of the foundational breath techniques used in the practice of kundalini yoga and is used as an energising and purifying breath. It is done by pumping the navel point in and out while breathing rapidly through the nose. It is always practised through the nostrils with the mouth closed. It releases toxins and deposits from the lungs, mucous linings, blood vessels and other cells, as well as expanding the lung capacity. There are lots of videos online where you can see it being done. However, it is not advised for menstruating women, people who suffer from dizziness, epilepsy, high blood pressure, heart disease, strokes or stomach ulcers.

The best thing about this is you can practise most of your breathing exercises pretty much anywhere without anyone noticing. Patients have told me they've done it on the tube on the way to work. You could easily do the same, or practise while driving, walking or simply chilling out in front of the TV.

EXERCISE

Exercise releases endorphins, the 'feel-good' chemicals in the brain, and gives us a natural high and boosts energy. Any form of exercise is good, from walking, to tennis or yoga. Walking or other exercise for half an hour a day is well recognised now as being as effective in treating mild to moderate depression as taking antidepressants.[6] The World Health Organization (WHO) recommends doing half an hour of exercise, five days a week.[7]

EAT TO COMBAT STRESS

Below are my recommendations for eating right to combat stress.

- *Junk food and takeaways are a far cry from a balanced and healthy diet.* They contain high levels of protein, fats and carbohydrates but without vital minerals and vitamins, causing stress on the body. Reducing stress is all about getting a balance of the correct vitamins and minerals, so I highly recommend avoiding all fast foods and takeaways as much as possible or only having them once a week.
- *Avoid tea, coffee and energy drinks when you're stressed.* They may appear refreshing when you're tired, but they also contain neuro-stimulators like caffeine and theobromine, which are proven to heighten stress. Stress makes you anxious and further stimulation can heighten this anxiety and even cause insomnia.
- *Soft drinks are packed full of useless calories and contain no vitamins or minerals.* When stressed, a build-up of carbon dioxide and lactates in the body can result in a condition called 'acidosis' (see page 82), which is damaging to health. The high levels of carbon dioxide in drinks aggravate stress.
- *Sugar should be avoided whenever possible.* Stress causes an increase in blood glucose levels which can lead to a higher risk of developing diabetes.
- *Reduce stress by eating fresh fruit and vegetables as they provide stress-reducing vitamins and minerals.* Vegetables also have a high fibre content, helpful in treating constipation – another long-term effect of stress.

- *Oily fish such as mackerel contain omega fatty acids which are extremely good for the heart, reducing the risk of heart disease.* Fish also contains choline – a great memory booster, which can help during period of stress.
- *Yoghurts provide minerals including calcium.* Calcium is essential for maintaining well-functioning nerve impulses. It can also be found in leafy green vegetables and avocados.
- *Flowers such as dandelion, chamomile and passion flower also relax both the body and mind.* These can be taken in the form of herbal tea or supplements.

MEDITATION AND MINDFULNESS

More than 100 scientific studies have shown the benefits of meditation, from lowering blood pressure to restoring energy to improving sleep to helping people give up smoking. It's all about trying to quieten the internal dialogue that goes on inside our heads most of the time. You can learn this at a yoga class or by listening to a meditation CD or you can give it a go yourself by sitting comfortably with your eyes closed and trying to quieten your mind. A good way to try this is to count as high as you can before your thoughts distract you. Most people rarely get above three so try not to feel frustrated. It's normal to have thoughts floating in. Just allow them to come in and out, pushing them away if necessary and start again.

Tonight when you brush your teeth, instead of letting your mind wander, spend some time focusing on the brushing, the sensations you feel and the sounds around you. This is a technique called mindfulness. It is simply being present in the moment and engaging the senses. You can try this whenever you are doing anything routine, from washing up to having a shower.

Energising meditation

Here is an example of an energising meditation that you can try right now to boost your energy. It can sometimes take a couple of weeks of regular practice to feel the full benefits of this. In this meditation, you use a combination of relaxation and mindfulness to lift your mood and energy levels.

- **Adopt an upright position.** Ensure that your back is relatively straight and your chest is open with shoulders back. Having a particularly open, erect, dignified posture can really help to energise you.
- **Take three deep in- and out-breaths.** Really feel those breaths moving in and out of your body.
- **Place one hand on your chest and one hand on your belly.** On your next in-breath, ensure that you breathe into your belly. The hand on your chest needs to remain relatively still, if possible.
- **Breathe out slowly from your mouth.** Feel the physical sensation as you do so.
- **Imagine yourself being energised as you breathe in.** If you're a visual person, imagine light entering into your body, nourishing all your cells with soothing, uplifting energy. If this isn't working for you, choose whatever image does work – there is no right or wrong.
- **Keep a light smile on your face throughout this energising breath meditation,** even if you don't really feel that happy, Doing so can help to boost your energy.
- **Guide your attention back each time your mind wanders.** Do so with kindness and gentleness and try not to get angry or frustrated with yourself.
- **Bring the meditation to a close after ten minutes or so.** Slowly open your eyes.

Gratitude and body scan meditation

This meditation is based on the body scan exercise. The aim is to focus your attention on individual parts of your body and try to release some muscle tension. It is best to start with the head and then work down through your face, throat, arms, chest, stomach, hips and legs. You then use gratitude after you're feeling more grounded to reduce your negative viewpoints and boost energy levels.

- **Lie down on your back in a warm, quiet place.** If that's not comfortable, whatever position that works for you is fine.
- **Feel your own natural breathing.** Notice the physical sensation of each breath, mindfully.
- **Begin scanning the physical sensation in your body, starting with your head.**
- **Become aware of any tension in each body part. Imagine your breath going into and out of the tension to soothe the tightness.** If the tension doesn't leave, that's okay – just be aware of the sensation and move on to the next part of your body.
- **Think about things for which you're grateful.** What's going well in your life? Perhaps remember that at least you've got this book and have made time to practise this meditation. Spend a couple of minutes reflecting on this reality.
- **End this meditation with three deep, mindful breaths.** Slowly stand up and have a good stretch before getting on with the rest of your day or evening.

Becoming more aware can help distract us from our internal chatter and produce a clearer mind. This will reduce stress and help you make better decisions.

EMOTIONAL FREEDOM TECHNIQUES

Emotional Freedom Techniques (EFT) can be used to overcome all sorts of physical and emotional health problems. It was founded by Gary Craig in 1993 and works on the principle that the cause of all negative emotions is a disruption in the body's energy system. It has been recognised by conventional medicine as having positive effects on conditions like post-traumatic stress disorder, depression and addiction (such as helping people to stop smoking).

EFT is a simplified form of acupuncture combined with parts of neuro-linguistic programming (NLP); that is, tapping on acupuncture points while saying specific phrases and affirmations that describe the problem you wish to address and release.

Conditions EFT can alleviate:

- addictions
- fatigue
- anger
- pain
- anxiety
- panic attacks
- cravings
- phobias
- depression
- unresolved emotional trauma

HOW TO USE EFT

There are plenty of great therapists specialising in EFT and lots of great websites too, but here's a mini-version you can use right now.

Step 1: It's best to be alone and uninterrupted when performing the EFT sequence. Think about the problem you wish to resolve and create a short problem statement that describes it. It should be personal to you and in your own words. Examples can be:

- I'm so tired
- I'm angry with Jessica
- I'm useless
- I'm unlovable
- I'm lonely
- I'm worried about money
- I'm terrified of dogs
- I want to give up smoking

Step 2: Create a longer problem statement based on this phrase: 'Even though I feel [insert your problem statement here], I deeply love and accept myself, without judgement. For example, 'Even though I feel *so tired*, I deeply love and accept myself without judgement.'

Step 3: Notice how severe this problem feels, rating its intensity from 1 to 10. Then notice where in the body you feel this problem, i.e. in your chest, stomach, etc. Notice if it has a particular feel to it, like a heaviness or sharpness, and if it has a size, shape or colour.

Step 4: Start tapping on the points below in sequence, beginning on the top of the head, working down the face and on to the chest and axilla (under your arm) and the fingertips. The tapping points are outlined in the illustration on page 166, courtesy of Andy

Bryce, EFT Master. Practitioners suggest tapping an average of seven times on each point, but this is not fixed and do not fixate on the number if it is going to cause you worry. Keep repeating the cycle until you feel the problem is less prominent than before.

When I'm out and about and feel stressed, I find it helpful to tap on my karate chop (outside edge of my hand below the little finger) or on my fingers to change my state.[8, 9]

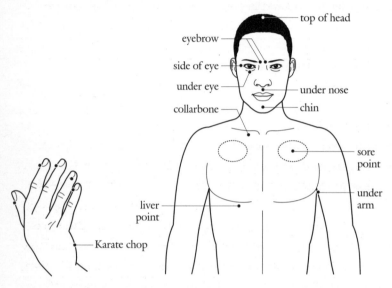

Emotional Freedom Technique (EFT) Tapping Points

GET HAPPY

My dad is the most serene person you'll ever meet, despite working about 80 hours a week and being in his sixties. He is never ill and has the blood pressure and arterial age of a 25-year-old. Is this just a coincidence? I don't think so. A review of over 160 studies showed 'clear and compelling' evidence that happy people tend to live longer and have better health than unhappy people.[10] Have you noticed that when you feel really happy you also feel really full of energy?

But what if you don't feel happy? Using affirmations and focusing on the good things in your life and the good qualities you have as a person can help. Examples of affirmations are: 'I am a good person who deserves good things', 'I love and accept myself unconditionally' and 'I have so much to offer'.

You can use whatever words you like as long as they resonate with you. Keep a list of 20 things you like about yourself and 20 things you have accomplished in your life so far. Keep this list close to you to remind yourself of your good qualities whenever you feel a little down. We all have good qualities, we just need reminding of them from time to time.

LAUGHTER IS THE BEST MEDICINE

Studies have shown that laughter has beneficial effects on the immune system by reducing stress and in turn improving natural killer (NK) cell activity. NK cells are a type of white blood cell and are key to a healthy immune system. Low NK cells are linked to decreased disease resistance and increased morbidity in people with cancer and HIV. The studies have shown laughter has a lowering effect on levels of adrenaline and noradrenaline and therefore would help with improving adrenal fatigue. Cortisol, the stress hormone, has immunosuppressive effects so there's some thought that laughter can act as an antidote to enhance the immune system in this way. There have also been studies that show laughter helps decrease the heart rate, breathing rate and blood pressure.[11] Obviously, it's hard to measure the true effects of laughter on stress and health as it can be quite subjective.

I laugh every day. I know I'm lucky because I naturally see the funny side of life and surround myself with light-hearted people. My favourite celebrities are all comedic in some way. If I'm not seeing my mates and sharing funny tales, I watch an episode of *Friends* or another funny TV show. I also like to remember amusing things that have happened to me or stories my friends have told me to bring up an instant supply of laughs.

I recommend you do the same, or find other ways to create your wellspring of joy and laughter.

LOVING RELATIONSHIPS

Have you ever had that feeling of new love or a crush, and suddenly you are full of energy despite having no sleep and feel fantastic and happy and no task is too mundane or dull? No man (or woman) is an island. We need loving relationships in our lives and to feel valued and loved to help support us, pick us up when we are down and to share good times and bad. Research has shown that good social relationships have a positive benefit on our mental and physical health. The most important type of relationships were found to be between a parent and child, and then in old age, probably because we are at our most vulnerable when we are very young or elderly. But loving relationships throughout all stages of our lives have a positive impact. Being married, having children or ties to a religious/spiritual or other organisation have all been shown to have favourable benefits on health.[12] Of course having a supportive, loving partner is ideal, but we can get love from other sources like friends and family too.

It's important to give as much warmth and love to the people already in your life, and to those you meet. Once you start living life in this way, you will receive lots of love back – that's how the universe works.

FEELING FULFILLED

When I'm at work and really enjoying myself, at a gig caught up in the euphoria of live music or spending a night with fabulous friends, I don't feel tired. When I get up in the morning and feel the work I'm going to do is worthwhile, I can get out of bed with a spring in my step. It's important to be doing something that makes you inspired to get out of bed, no matter how little sleep you've had.

The fantastic book *Healthy at 100* by John Robbins looks at the populations of South America, Central America and Japan where people routinely live until they're over 100 years old. The studies have shown common trends: these populations all have a mainly plant-based diet; the older people still work and do physical exercise; they live with family; and are respected and valued members of society.[13] This just proves how important it is to feel valued and believe you make a contribution to the world.

I love my work, but it took me a long time to find a career that truly feeds my soul. I know how it feels to not want to go to work and feel like you aren't making a difference. If you can't find work that nourishes you, then make it your goal to look for interests outside of work which fulfil you. Find an inspiring life goal. Examples of this could be doing volunteer work like helping a neighbour or a local organisation. Think about what you love. So if you enjoy music, think about joining a band or choir or get involved in organising charity gigs. If you're excited about drama join a local acting club. If you love children, think about volunteering at a children's home or do some babysitting. There are loads of charity excursions you could get involved with to raise money for different charities, such as trekking up Mount Kilimanjaro or along the Inca Trail or the Great Wall of China. You would get fit, raise money for a cause, meet new people and have a life-changing experience. It requires a lot of discipline and hard work to achieve a challenging goal. And having the inspiration to work towards something you believe in provides a constant source of energy and motivation. The world is out there and waiting for you – go get it!

ACTION PLAN

Now that you know stress is as bad for your health as smoking and decreases your energy levels, find a way to de-stress that works for you. It is important to remember to appreciate what you have already and to find something in your life that makes you feel fulfilled. Emotional energy drainers need to be addressed, such as avoiding people who make you feel negative about yourself and finding ways to replenish your emotional energy by taking time out, doing hobbies you enjoy and finding some inner peace.

CHAPTER 12
SUPPLEMENTING YOUR HEALTH

Almost one in three people in the UK takes a vitamin supplement,[1] but, as a general rule, I believe *everyone* needs to take supplements in some shape or form. There are undoubtedly mixed feelings about this topic and people often ask me why I advocate taking them as research hasn't always supported their benefits. This also accompanies a very common statement, *'I prefer to get my vitamins from my food.'* My response is always, *'So you eat at least five portions of fruit and vegetables a day, every day then?'* More often than not the answer is a sheepish 'no'. If someone is really interested I tell them some of the information I've outlined for you below, but if not I just leave it, as no one likes a bore at a cocktail party banging on about fruit and vegetables.

Here's why I feel we need supplementation in addition to a healthy diet:

- The majority of people simply don't eat enough fruit and vegetables. The World Health Organization recommends we have five portions of fruit and vegetables a day. In Australia, their recommendation is seven a day (two fruit and five vegetables) and in Japan it's 12. The majority of the population in the UK don't even make the lower limit recommendation of five a day. In fact, it's believed only one in seven of us actually achieves our five a day. All our vitamins and minerals are found in natural foods, not in the processed foods that make up the majority of our diets. Supplements are no substitute for eating actual fruit and vegetables, but they do help to bridge the gap.

- Even those of us who do meet our five-a-day requirement may need supplements. In the days of our parents and grandparents, people would buy their fruit and vegetables from a local greengrocer. Moreover, the produce would have been grown in the local area and so hadn't travelled too far. Nowadays the majority of fruit and vegetables we buy in the supermarkets come from abroad and are likely to have been picked months ago, meaning the nutritional value will have depleted over time. Most fruit and vegetables have been preserved with pesticides and other chemicals to help them grow, been mass produced and travelled from the other side of the world. This means that we're ingesting large amounts of chemicals and our bodies need support in removing these toxins from our systems. This is why buying local and organic produce where possible is far better.

- In general, the quality of fruit and vegetables is not the same as it once was. Donald Davis and his team of researchers from the University of Texas (UT) studied US Department of Agriculture nutritional data from both 1950 and 1999 for 43 different vegetables and fruits. Their landmark study found that levels of protein, calcium, phosphorus, iron, riboflavin (vitamin B2) and vitamin C have declined over the past half century. Davis and his colleagues put this down to the shifting focus of agricultural practices away from nutrition and towards improving traits such as size, growth rate and pest resistance.[2]

- Over the years, the soil we use has also become depleted of nutrients. Fruit and vegetables grown decades ago were much richer in vitamins and minerals than the varieties most of us get today. The main culprit in this trend is soil depletion. The fertilisers and chemicals used in the soil mean that crops grow faster and bigger, but there's an increasing lack of the trace minerals needed to keep our fruit and vegetables full of goodness. In fact, a Kushi Institute analysis of nutrient data from 1975 to 1997 found that average calcium levels in 12 fresh vegetables dropped 27 per cent, iron levels 37 per cent, vitamin A levels 21 per cent and vitamin C levels 30 per cent. A similar study of British nutrient data from 1930 to 1980 found that in 20 vegetables the average calcium content had declined 19 per cent, iron 22 per cent and potassium 14 per cent. Yet another study concluded that one person would have to eat eight oranges today to derive the same amount of vitamin A as someone from our grandparents' generation would have received from one.[3]

This is the reason I recommend everybody should take a *good-quality multivitamin*. I normally recommend getting one from a health-food shop or from a specialist company as opposed to a supermarket. The reason for this is because more expensive multivitamins usually contain more absorbable forms of nutrients, so it's not always cost effective to go for the very cheapest. Some of the cheaper products also contain synthetic inactive ingredients or colours and preservatives which means that it won't be absorbed by the body.

DO MULTIVITAMINS REALLY WORK?

Three recent studies published in the journal *Annals of Internal Medicine* concluded that research doesn't show a health benefit to taking most vitamin supplements, and that they don't seem to prevent death or disease. The studies published looked for improved cognitive functioning in men, the potential benefits of multivitamins in people who've had a heart attack[4] and the effects of vitamin and mineral supplements in preventing cancer and heart disease.[5] Based on that, you may be wondering why *I'm* advocating supplements?

Firstly, what most people don't know is that the studies above had high drop-out rates – almost half in one study, in fact – and we don't know the dietary history of the participants. It would be far more useful to see a study that looked into things such as if a person gets more or fewer viral illnesses than the average person who doesn't take multivitamins and what their energy levels are like.

Professor Balz Frei, director at the Linus Pauling Institute at Oregon State University, says the methods of these studies, which try to measure the effects of micronutrients like they are powerful prescription drugs, are flawed. He says that the studies need to do a baseline analysis to identify nutritional inadequacies and then need to see if supplementation remedies the inadequacies. In the USA, 90 per cent of adults don't get the required amounts of vitamins D and E for health, 40 per cent don't get enough vitamin C and half don't get enough vitamin A, calcium and magnesium according to Frei's research. UK research has shown similar results with an estimation that 70–80 per cent of the population will have insufficient vitamin D levels. Smokers, the obese, ill, injured or elderly often have an elevated need for vitamins and minerals.

There are also several flaws in vitamin C research. In cell culture experiments, which are often conducted in high oxygen environments, vitamin C is unstable and can actually appear harmful. In addition, animal studies aren't accurate as most animals, unlike humans, can synthesise their own vitamin C and don't need to obtain it from their diet. This makes most animal studies about vitamin C irrelevant to humans.

The longest and largest clinical studies looking at vitamin/ mineral supplements found a huge reduction in cancer and cataracts in male physicians over 50 years old. This study suggested that if every adult in the USA took vitamin/mineral supplements it could prevent up to 130,000 cases of cancer each year. This benefit would be in addition to providing basic good health by supporting normal functioning of the body, growth and metabolism.[6]

Of course it would be wonderful if we could get the majority of our nutrition from the food we eat, but a multivitamin in conjunction with a healthy diet helps to bridge this gap and can help to improve our health and energy levels.

If you want to take a supplement, firstly do some research and find a reputable company who are committed to research and evaluation of their products, or alternatively take a wholefood supplement. Pick a product in an easier-to-absorb capsule form and be prepared to have to take more than one tablet a day, as it's hard to cram all the vitamins and minerals you need into just one tablet.

WHAT TO AVOID

It's better to spend a little more on multivitamins and avoid cheaper versions that contain sugar, lactose, artificial colours and flavours and other non-nutritional substances. Cheaper brands also use lower-quality excipients, which are non-nutritional substances that bind each tablet together, which means the vitamin tablets won't be as well absorbed or as useful to the body. Also, lower-quality supplements use below-par nutrients, such as magnesium oxide, which are not as well absorbed. If your multivitamin contains magnesium oxide it's probably not good quality.

Reasons to take a multivitamin

- The food we eat is nutritionally depleted
- Most people don't eat the minimum of five a day
- Multivitamins will help us deal with pollution and stress
- Even if you eat well, supplements will help your system run even more effectively

---

WHOLEFOOD SUPPLEMENTS

I take wholefood supplements, which means that the vitamins and minerals come from a food source. It's thought that these compounds are better absorbed than synthetic forms. We all know that wholefoods are better than refined foods. There have never been any arguments that honey is a better choice for you than white sugar or that brown rice is better than white rice. Should the same theory not be used for supplements too?

In synthetic supplements there are only isolated vitamins present. Wholefood supplements contain vitamins as well as a variety of enzymes, coenzymes, antioxidants, trace elements, activators and other unknown factors that all work together synergistically, so that the vitamin complex can work in your body more effectively.

There are greens formulas, and other fruit and vegetable blends available, as well as natural vitamin C formulas made from

The National Institute for Health and Care Excellence (Nice) recommendations for people to take vitamin supplements

Although a lot of doctors think that supplements are not needed, the following people are recommended to take vitamins routinely. In addition, I think anyone with chronic illness or a health condition should take supplementation regularly.

- Pregnant or breast-feeding women
- Children aged six months to four years old
- Vitamin D for those aged 65 years old, children aged six months until five years old and pregnant and breast-feeding women

fruits rich in vitamin C that may work more in synergy with your body than synthetic formulations. See the Resources section on pages 239–40 for more information or speak to a nutritionist for more advice.

OMEGA-3 FISH OIL

Another supplement I recommend for everybody is an omega fish oil capsule. Omega-3 and -6 fish oils are also called essential fatty acids (EFAs), because they can't be produced by the body but are essential for it to function healthily. They can be naturally obtained in the diet from oily fish such as mackerel, sardines, tuna, herring and salmon. It is important to note that there are vegetarian and vegan forms of omega-3 oils made from plant origin available which have all the same great benefits. Please see the Resources section on pages 239–40 for more guidance.

- It's believed that the EFAs work from inside the membranes of cells and may help to improve the heart's electrical activity and blood pressure. Other studies have shown that omega-3 fish oils protect against strokes and some forms of cancer.
- Omega-3 fish oils boost energy by providing healthy fats for the body that are released slowly to maintain energy levels. They are also powerful antioxidants that boost the immune system and fight fatigue.
- Omega-3 fish oils are thought to help improve memory, coordination, dyslexia, bipolar disorder and depression. They help improve electrical function between nerves and are essential for healthy brain conduction.
- A good balance of omega-6 and omega-3 fish oils has a beneficial effect on asthma.
- Fish oils have shown additional benefits such as preventing Alzheimer's disease, inflammation in the body and diabetes and help with weight management.

Taking an omega-3 supplement will help redress the balance between omega-6 and the levels of omega-3 in the body. A ratio of omega-6 to omega-3 of 1:1 to 4:1 has the most beneficial effect on the body. In Western diets our ratio of omega-6 to omega-3 is approximately 15:1. Too much omega-6 and not enough omega-3 increases inflammation within the body, which in turn contributes to illness and feeling unwell and fatigued.

DO OMEGA-3 FISH OILS CAUSE PROSTATE CANCER?

There was some controversy in 2013 about a study that claimed that taking omega-3 fish oils increased the risk of getting prostate cancer in men.[7] The study showed that men with a higher blood concentration of omega-3 fat had a 44 per cent increased risk of developing low-grade prostate cancer compared to those with lower levels. In previous studies, foods rich in omega-3 fats have previously been shown to *prevent* prostate cancer from spreading, and one meta-analysis study from 2010 showed that fish consumption was associated with a 63 per cent reduction in prostate cancer mortality.[8] In the controversial 2013 study in question, 53 per cent of the subjects with prostate cancer were smokers, 64 per cent regularly consumed alcohol and 80 per cent were overweight or obese. Several previous studies have shown that obesity or being overweight increases the risk of prostate cancer.[9]

VITAMIN D

I also recommend taking a vitamin D supplement. Vitamin D is actually a hormone synthesised by the body from sunlight, and is essential for keeping bones and muscles strong and healthy. Even a mild lack of vitamin D can cause muscle aches, tiredness and general pains. However, there's very little vitamin D in our food, only a small amount in egg yolks, oily fish, liver and wild mushrooms. We need sunlight to make vitamin D, and it's thought that 15 minutes a day of sun exposure to the arms and legs in Caucasian skin is enough to get the recommended amount. People with darker skin may require 30 minutes a day. In both cases, avoid wearing sunscreen, at least for the allocated time, in order to absorb the vitamin D effectively. In the UK especially, we simply don't get enough sunlight to synthesise sufficient vitamin-D levels. Therefore we're all at risk of being deficient. Supplements need to be in the form of D3 to be best absorbed. It is recommended that we take between 600–800 IU (international units) a day but I recommend taking 1000 IU.

In addition to these three basics (multivitamins, Omega 3 oil, vitamin D), most people require extra supplementation in some form:

ANTIOXIDANTS

These are essential for boosting the immune system which keeps the body healthy and energised and also keeps you looking young – both on the inside and on the outside. Let me give you some examples of how antioxidants work:

- When you get sunburnt, your skin needs to heal from the damage the sun has caused. Antioxidants play a role in this process.
- When you eat certain foods, they can cause inflammation in the stomach and this needs to be repaired by antioxidants.
- When we smoke or drink alcohol, we use antioxidants to repair the damage, which is one of the reasons why smokers and heavy alcohol users look older than their years because there are not enough antioxidants to cope with the stress the body is under.

Examples of antioxidants are vitamins C and E. I take extra antioxidant supplements to keep me looking young on the outside, but to also get the beneficial effects on the inside. Antioxidants are in certain fruit and vegetables that we eat. The main way to identify this is that foods with vibrant colours are rich in antioxidants: think red cabbage, blueberries, dark green leafy vegetables, carrots and red cherries.

SUPERFOODS

There are some fantastic superfoods that you can add to your diet that are full of nutrients. Although technically there is no such thing as a 'superfood', these are so-called because they are high in vitamins and minerals and there have been huge health benefits claimed about them. The truth is, there are huge health benefits to eating all fruit and vegetables, but here are my favourite 'superfoods' that I regularly incorporate into my diet to boost my energy and overall health:

Wheatgrass is grown from wheat seeds, and contains a high amount of chlorophyll. Chlorophyll absorbs sunlight when it is grown and is a natural source of energy. It is also rich in protein, which boosts energy. Most people juice it, or add it to juices in powdered form, but it's also available in supplement form. It has high levels of chlorophyll and the Hippocrates Health Institute claims it has many health benefits such as stimulating the thyroid gland, increasing the red blood cell count, detoxifying the blood, liver and gastrointestinal tract and stimulating metabolism, reducing acidity in the body and relieving stomach ulcers, constipation, diarrhoea, ulcerative colitis and reducing the damaging effects of radiation.

Barley grass has similar benefits to wheatgrass, but is often better tolerated as wheatgrass can cause nausea in some people. Research by the Resource Research Association, Office of Science and Technology, and Japan Food Analysis Center showed dried barley grass juice has more sodium, calcium, magnesium, iron and copper phosphorus than spinach.

Spirulina is a form of blue-green algae and can be bought in powdered, tablet or capsule form. It's a form of protein and is a great energy booster, as well as being beneficial in easing sneezing from allergies, strengthens the immune system and helps control high blood pressure and cholesterol. It is rich in protein and amino acids and contains vitamin B12 which works to increase energy and helps with mental concentration. It is also a great detoxifier for the body. It has an excellent balance of nutrients including chlorophyll, carotenoids, vitamins, minerals, unique phytonutrients and all the essential amino acids to keep you energized all day. I find it gives me energy and also helps strengthen my nails and hair. It's generally safe but should be bought from a reliable supplier and choose organic wherever possible as it can be contaminated with heavy metals. It should also be avoided in those with severe seafood allergies, iodine allergies or hyperthyroidism.

Maca is from a Peruvian root and is rich in calcium, potassium, iron, phosphorus, magnesium, silica and zinc. It strengthens the body and increases stamina, and can boost energy levels. It also stabilises hormone levels and can relieve pre-menstrual tension and menopausal symptoms, as well as boosting sexual health. A study showed that sperm counts and motility were improved by men taking maca.

Co-Enzyme Q10 (CoQ10) is a vitamin-like substance found throughout the body, but especially in the heart, liver, kidney, and pancreas. It's eaten in small amounts in meat and seafood. It is responsible for generating the energy 'currency' of all the cells in the body, in the form of adenosine triphosphate (ATP). Simply put, your cells require CoQ10 to help produce the energy you need to live. It is also found abundantly in the mitochondria – the cells in our body that produce energy. CoQ10 also has powerful antioxidant and anti-ageing properties, as it helps reduce stress to your cells, and helps the tissues and organs and supports muscle recovery from intensive workouts and exercise. A research team from China also found that individuals placed on CoQ10 (300mg per day for 12 weeks) showed marked improvement in blood flow to the heart and improved energy within the artery cells. CoQ10 has also been proven to reduce heart failure and decrease mortality rates by a half. Our bodies produce less CoQ10 the older we get and it is also reduced by taking certain drugs like statins for cholesterol, so it needs to be replaced to improve health and energy. I would recommend taking CoQ10 as a supplement at a dose of 30–100mg a day. It comes in two forms, ubiquinol and ubiquinone, and I would recommend getting ubiquinol as it is easier for the body to absorb.

Alpha-lipoic acid is a fatty acid found naturally inside every cell in the body. It's needed by the body to produce energy for our body's normal functions. Alpha lipoic acid is also an antioxidant, and can neutralise potentially harmful chemicals called free radicals. What makes alpha lipoic acid unique is that it functions in water and fat, unlike the more common antioxidants vitamins C and E. Alpha lipoic acid also increases the formation of glutathione, an important antioxidant that helps the body eliminate potentially harmful substances.

Recent research has shown that the more chemicals we are exposed to – through our food, the products we use on our skin or our environment – the greater our chances of developing serious illnesses and conditions such as diabetes. Therefore taking this supplement will boost your body to help combat this. I would recommend taking alpha lipoic acid as a supplement 100–200mg once a day.

Ginseng is a natural energy booster. In fact, a study has shown that it can even improve the fatigue associated with chemotherapy in patients with cancer.[10] Other benefits of ginseng are improved memory, improved physical performance and aiding the body to cope with stress. There are many different types of ginseng, such as American, Red, Siberian, Chinese and Korean. These plants are considered to be 'adaptogens', which means they are a type of plant that helps mediate a metabolic process within the body and helps the body cope with stress. I personally take Korean ginseng.

A dose of between 200–500mg, one to two times a day is usually sufficient and safe for most people.

Hopefully this chapter will have increased your understanding of supplements and convinced you that by relying only on our natural diet to provide nutrients, we may struggle to meet our nutritional needs, as our food is becoming depleted and polluted. If you are low on energy, taking some of the supplements outlined above can help you feel less fatigued and boost your energy. Why not try them and see for yourself? There are many good-quality supplements out there and it's worth spending time researching companies for the best. Bear in mind it can take a few months to see the full effects of some supplements, but the effects of 'super-foods' like spirulina will be felt a lot quicker.

CHAPTER 13
MOVE

It is important to learn how to exercise and move your body to improve your health. Once you start to move, you will regain your energy and reduce the stress in your life.

The benefits of exercise are well documented and I am sure you are aware of the long-term effects exercise has on weight, heart disease, joints and your respiratory system. I have never heard anyone say that exercise is bad for you. No matter what your size is or what your medical conditions may be, there is an exercise that will suit you and help your condition.

However, what most people do not realise is that you don't have to run for an hour or do intense cardio workouts to stay fit and healthy. In fact, it has been documented that strenuous cardio workouts can cause joint damage and lead to arthritis in the future. We were not designed to run for an hour on a treadmill. It can be more damaging to do intensive exercise when you are already feeling weak and fatigued as this puts more strain on the adrenal glands. Our ancestors did not have to schedule time to exercise. It was part of daily life, so it's important that you find a way to incorporate movement into your everyday routine.

It can be so hard to find the motivation to exercise. When you feel tired it can be the last thing you want to do. I spoke to personal trainer Ollie Phillips about this problem, which is something he sees with his clients all the time. Ollie says that we need to adapt our mindset to get the most out of exercise. He says we live in a work culture: from the moment our alarm goes off in the morning our mindset is about getting out to work, to expend our time and efforts either for our own financial gain or that of our employer's. We can spend an average of 10–12 hours a day revolving our lives around work, but when it comes to doing 10 or 12 minutes of exercise we struggle to meet this simple task. It is obvious that after a long day of work, whether it's in the office or at home looking after children, we are going to feel tired. But Ollie says this is psychological rather than a physiological tiredness. He told me, 'The power of the mind is very strong, and it can determine whether or not we are going to follow through with a physiological task or stress. Exercise is simply physiological stress and can be very off-putting when we picture in our minds the blood, sweat and tears that some may go through in the gym environment.'

However, as already stated, we do not need to put ourselves through that amount of stress to achieve our health goals. We do not have to run on a treadmill for an hour to feel the benefits of exercise or lift ridiculously heavy weights. If we think about the intensity of activities on a scale of 1 to 10, reading this book would be about a 1, and doing a sprint as fast as you can for 50 yards would be a 10. Most people doing an exercise class or workout session work at a level of intensity between 5 to 8. If we do a brisk walk, the intensity would be a 5, and that is enough to cause a significant increase in energy within ourselves. We rarely reach a level above 5 during our work commute or by doing typical activities in an office. The simple fact is we need to specu-late to accumulate, meaning that we need to expend some energy in the form of exercise in order to feel more energetic. We have plenty of stored energy and gain a lot of energy from the food we consume, which means feeling too tired to exercise, despite our best intentions, is often more of a psychological tiredness than a physical one.

So get up and move! Start with 10 minutes a day if you are new to exercise and build it up by five minutes every week.

YOGA

The more I learn about yoga the more convinced I become about its health benefits for the body and the mind. Yoga has been proven to help aches and pains such as back pain, lower blood pressure, heart problems, depression and stress, as well as the obvious benefits of increased flexibility, body strength and balance.

Yoga can help to naturally improve energy. This is because yoga works to unblock energy that is stuck along the spine. Followers of yoga believe you are bringing 'prana' or your body's life force back into these areas through breathing and movement. Active yoga poses that help to gently stretch the spine as well as stimulate the blood flow are invigorating.

Here are some examples of restorative and energising yoga poses you can do:

CORPSE POSE

Corpse pose, also called savasana in Sanskrit, is one of the most relaxing yet energising poses in yoga. It's a great way to end your exercise session, or it can be used alone to regain tranquillity and focus.

1. Lie flat on your back with your feet hip-width apart and your arms slightly away from your sides, so air can circulate around your body.
2. Roll your shoulders down and back as you lengthen your neck.
3. Take a mental note of areas in your body that are holding tension as you take deep breaths and focus on relaxing your muscles.
4. Remain in this position for five to 30 minutes, while trying to keep your mind empty of all distractions.
5. Your palms should be facing upwards, as a signal of relinquishing and letting go of stress and emotion.

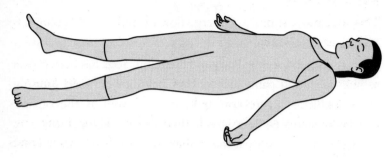

Corpse Pose – Shavasana

When lying in savasana, it is a good time to practise *ujjayi breathing*, or ocean breathing. Ujjayi breathing (pronounced ooh-jy, jy rhyming with pie) is a fundamental of yoga practice. It allows us to take in much more oxygen and 'prana' and switches us from the 'fight or flight' mode which occurs when the adrenal glands are under stress to a more relaxed state. It is the breath we naturally and eventually fall into when we are asleep.

To learn how to do this type of breathing, inhale through your nose and then exhale slowly through an open mouth. Direct your exhale via the back of the throat so it makes a 'ha' sound. Repeat this several times, and then try it again but this time with your mouth closed. Direct the breath from the back of the throat to the nose. This should make a soft hissing sound. The importance of this breath is to slow the breathing down, allow you to monitor the evenness of the breath and cause the mind to focus on the breath and to stop wandering. Ideally, this should be done for five to eight minutes to begin with, before building it up to 10 to 15 minutes of practice. When you are finished return to your normal breathing for a few minutes. Yogis believe that we can detox through the lungs as well as via the skin in sweat, urination and defecation, and this is a good way to start this process.

ARM PUMPS

This yoga move stimulates energy flow from the spinal column to other parts of the body.

1. Interlace your fingers and clasp hands with your knuckles facing out and palms facing in.
2. Extend your arms forward, then inhale as you bring your arms up over your head. Exhale as your lower your hands down to your knees.
3. Continue this motion with each strong breath, inhaling and lifting your arms then exhaling as you lower them down. You can start by doing this move for 1–2 minutes, and work up to 5 minutes.

CAT POSE/COW POSE

The cat pose is often paired with the cow pose creating a rejuvenating sequence. These poses increase flexibility to the spine, as well as stretch the back of the torso and neck. They also softly stimulate the abdominal organs.

1. Begin on your hands and knees, with your wrists directly under your shoulders, and your knees placed directly under

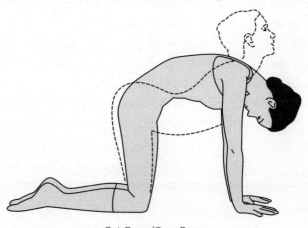

Cat Pose/Cow Pose

your hips. Place your knees hip-distance apart and centre your head and neck in a neutral position.

2. To begin the cow pose, inhale as you drop your stomach towards the mat or floor. Lift your chin and chest, as you gaze up towards the ceiling.

3. As you exhale, draw your belly button up towards your spine and round your back toward the ceiling – simulating a cat stretching its back – to complete cat pose. Relax your neck and allow your head to lower towards the floor.

4. Repeat this move for 1–2 minutes as you inhale into cow pose, and exhale into cat pose.

LYING TWISTS

Yoga twists can squeeze out the anxiety and frustrations of your day, similar to wringing out a sponge. Twists also stimulate and detoxify the organs of your torso.

1. Lie on your back with your knees bent and your feet flat on the floor. Extend your arms out to each side, keeping your shoulder blades on the floor.

2. Exhale as you drop your knees to the left and gently turn your head to the right. Keep your shoulder blades pressing towards the floor. Allow the force of gravity to drop your knees even closer to the floor.

3. Hold this pose for several breaths, then inhale as you slowly bring your knees back to your chest.

4. Exhale as you release your legs to the right.

5. Repeat 3–5 times on both sides.

BACK BENDS – BRIDGE POSE

The bridge pose improves fatigue, anxiety and insomnia. It can also improve headaches, backaches and digestion.

1. Lying on your back, bend your knees and press both feet flat on to the floor with your arms on the floor to your side.

2. Lift your hips up as high as possible and breathe deeply for five breaths and then drop your hips to the floor gently.

3. Repeat this three to five times.

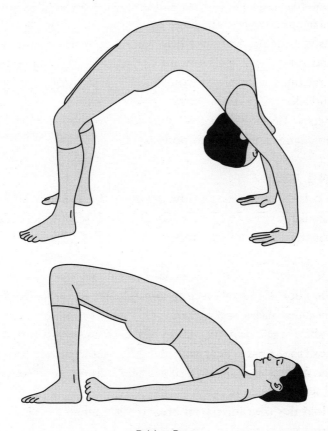

Bridge Pose

HALF SUN SALUTATION (SURYA NAMASKARA)

This is a great pose to do first thing in the morning to boost your energy.

1. To start the sequence, stand up straight with your feet together and arms by your sides with open palms.

2. Sweep the arms up and extend them over your head on the inhalation of the breath, then exhale and bow forwards into a forward bend.

3. On the next inhale lift the torso halfway up, placing your hands on your shins, or the calves if that is too difficult. Fold forwards again on the exhale.

4. When you inhale sweep back up again and bring your palms together into a prayer position. Repeat this sequence three to five times.

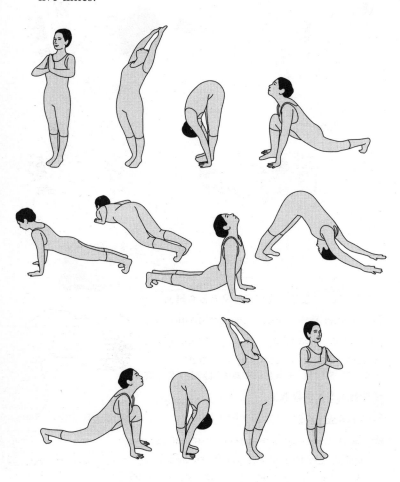

Half Sun Salutation – Surya Namaskara

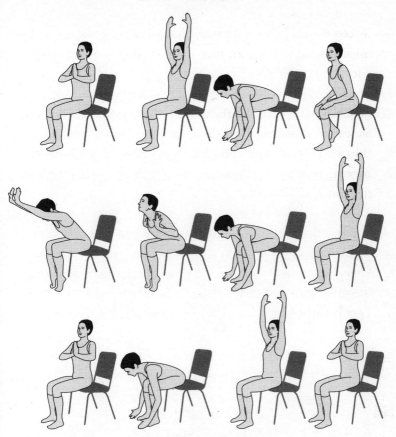

Half Sun Salutation – Modified (easier) version for those with mobility problems

CAMEL POSE (USTRASANA)

The camel pose opens up the front of the body, expanding the chest and the lungs as well as stretching the spine.

1. Kneel down with your legs straight behind you.
2. Lean backwards and rest your hands either on the lower back, or reach down to touch the heels if you can manage it.

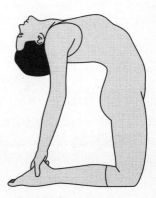

Camel Pose – Ustrasana

If you find it hard to unwind in the evening, it might help you to try the following yoga poses.

THE FORWARD BEND (PASCHIMOTTANASANA)

1. Sit on the floor with your bottom supported with a folded blanket or firm cushion and your legs straight in front of you.
2. Press actively through to your heels. Make sure your weight is even on both buttocks.
3. Turn the tops of the thighs in slightly and press them down into the floor. Keep your hands beside you and press them into the floor.
4. Bend forwards as much as you can comfortably. Rest your hands on your legs or the floor if you cannot reach.
5. Take breaths and move forwards as much as you can. Rest in this pose for one to three minutes.
6. To move out of this pose first lift the torso away from the thighs, straighten the arms and then lift up on the inhale.

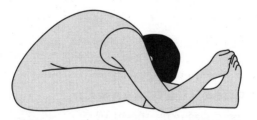

The Forward Bend – Paschimottanasana

CHILD'S POSE (BAKASANA)

This is a relaxing pose and can be done from anywhere between 30 seconds or a few minutes.

1. Kneel on the floor, keep your big toes together and sit on your heels. Widen the knees about as wide as your hips.

2. Exhale and lay your torso between your thighs. Lengthen your tail bone and stretch your neck to try and separate the base of the skull from the back of the neck.
3. Lay your hands on the floor alongside your torso with the palms up. Try and release your shoulders towards the floor.

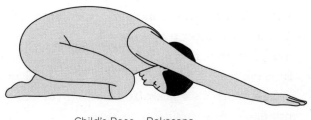

Child's Pose – Bakasana

EXTENDED PUPPY POSE (UTTANA SHISHOSANA)

1. Come on to all fours, making sure your hips are above your knees and your wrists are in line with your shoulders.
2. Exhale and move your buttocks halfway back towards your heels.
3. Keep your arms strong but do not allow your elbows to touch the ground. Lengthen your back and try and bring your head down to touch the ground if possible.
4. Press the hands down and stretch through the arms while pulling your hips back toward your heels.

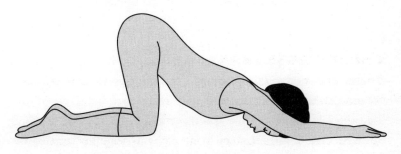

Extended Puppy Pose – Uttana Shishosana

BUTTERFLY POSE, WITH THE HEAD COMING DOWN TOWARDS THE FEET

The benefits of this pose are to stretch the spine and the hamstrings. If you have back pains or aren't that flexible then this pose is best done by sitting on a cushion so the knees are below the hips.

1. From a seated position, bring the soles of your feet together and then slide them away from you.
2. Allow your back to round, fold forwards and lightly rest your hands on your feet or on the floor. Your head should hang down towards your heels. You can support your head with your hands if the strain is too much.
3. If your back is feeling pressure then you can keep your feet together and lie down.
4. Try and hold for 10–20 seconds, repeat 3–5 times.

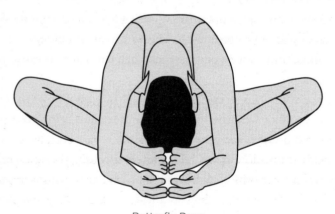

Butterfly Pose

Kundalini yoga is a form of yoga that works to help move energy around the body. It combines physical postures, stretching, breathing, meditation, mantra and relaxation. It is based on the principle that everyone has the energy of kundalini flowing through their bodies, but in many cases it becomes trapped or reduced due to the stresses of daily life. Regular practice of this sort of yoga works to release the dormant energy in our bodies. This energy is stimulated to rise up the spinal column and activate the pineal gland in the brain. Once this happens, we can use the energy of the body and mind properly, rather than being controlled by our emotions. There are many great videos online and DVDs to learn more about kundalini yoga (see Resources section on pages 239–40) or look for a class in your local area.

Yoga has beneficial effects on the mind as well as the body. Other forms of exercise that are both gentle and good for you are walking and swimming. Research has shown that walking for half an hour a day is as beneficial on your mood as taking an antidepressant in cases of mild or moderate depression. The most important thing is to find something you enjoy and therefore will do regularly. For example, I am not much of a gym-goer and find it hard to make time to go, but love to dance to my favourite songs. This is something I can do for 10 minutes in my living room so no excuse for me not to do it! Perhaps find a class of some sort to go to if you are low on motivation.

ACHES AND PAINS

The more tired you are, the more aches and pains you have. When the body is run-down physically and emotionally, your pain receptors are more sensitive. Aches and pains are also major symptoms of conditions where tiredness is a feature, such as chronic fatigue syndrome, fibromyalgia and anaemia.

A lot of us suffer from aches and pains in the shoulder area or back. In general, this is caused mainly by having excess weight or not being active enough. I know that for myself, after I sit all day or spend long periods driving, the aches in my shoulders and neck are worse. Many people come to their GP about this problem, when in reality this is probably the worst person to see. Doctors have very little training in muscular problems, and in my opinion you would be better off seeing an osteopath, chiropractor or someone who specialises in muscular aches and pains.

I would recommend the following tools as essential to help with your aches and pains: a foam roller and tennis balls. A foam roller is very useful to help aches and pains in the lower back, hip and leg areas. It can also be used to realign the spine, by lying on it vertically (see illustrations that follow). Foam rollers are available in most sports shops or online and can be bought for as little as £10. Tennis balls can be used to massage the deep tissues (or fascia) in the neck and shoulder areas. Lie on them and move slowly up and down or in a circular motion. They can be used on all areas of the body, and the foam roller can be used in a similar way. This is called a myo-fascial release. I would do this at least twice a day to begin with for five to ten minutes, especially if you have areas of tension or pain.

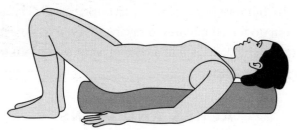

Foam Rolling – to support and release tension in the spine

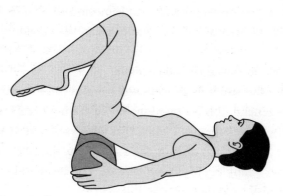

Foam Rolling – to ease muscle tension in the lower back, buttocks and hips

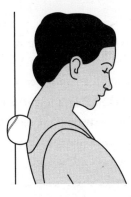

Using tennis balls to perform a myofascial release in the shoulders

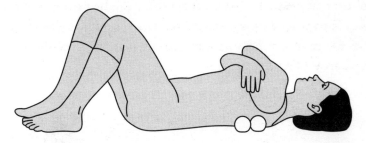

Using tennis balls to perform a myofascial release in the shoulders

The reason we have so much muscular tension is because we just don't use our bodies enough. It really is a case of 'use it or lose it'. Compare the way a five-year-old runs with how an 80-year-old moves. A five-year-old runs crazily, moving all parts of their body, with no fear. A five-year-old can put their foot in their mouth! Then slowly, over time we lose this ability to move so freely. We stop running for fun, jumping and skipping. Our muscles get weak, but more importantly the fascia, which is the deep tissues between the muscles, gets stiff. Most of the pain we experience is due to the fascia, not the muscles. The majority of 80-year-olds are unable to walk unaided or bend down for this reason.

ACTION PLAN

Just get moving. We spend all our time sat down at work, in the car or sat on the sofa watching *EastEnders*! Get moving and you will reap the benefits in later years. One of my favourite quotes by Edward Stanley, the Earl of Derby from 1826–93, is 'Those who don't have time for exercise, will sooner or later have to make time for illness.' Even five minutes is better than nothing. Also remember that exercise can be a walk, and try and incorporate it into your routine as much as possible – use the stairs, park far away in the supermarket, cycle to work. There are lots of good exercise DVDs available or videos on YouTube so if you are a busy person you can do a quick workout at home any time of day that is convenient for you. I know what a struggle this is when you are busy, but you can do it, just get creative!

CHAPTER 14
BIO-IDENTICAL HORMONES

It has become a more frequent occurrence in my medical practice to see middle-aged women who are extremely tired. Some of these still feel fatigued even after following my guidelines on eating, managing their weight and exercising. This was rather baffling until I discovered the missing piece of the puzzle: bio-identical hormones.

Bio-identical hormones can be used for women who are having menopausal problems, and other female problems like premenstrual tension, fibroids and even migraines. Balancing hormones can be a way to improve energy, vitality, concentration and mood.

WHAT ARE BIO-IDENTICAL HORMONES?

A bio-identical hormone has the same chemical and molecular structure as the hormones made naturally by the body. This means that bio-identical hormones are 100 per cent identical to the chemical structure of oestrogen, progesterone and testosterone produced by the human body. These naturally occurring hormones are sourced from plants like wild yams and soya beans and manufactured by pharmaceutical companies into lozenges to be taken by mouth or cream forms. They are often called 'natural' as they originate from plant sources. Their chemical structure is the same as the body's natural hormones, but they still go through a pharmaceutical process to compound them into lozenges or creams.

So, bio-identical hormone replacement therapy (BHRT) is the precise use of hormones to replace and rebalance the body's natural hormones during the changes that lead up to menopause and andropause (the hormonal changes in men). BHRT can also be used as a treatment to balance hormonal conditions such as premenstrual tension, painful and heavy periods, fibroids, endometriosis, post-natal depression and other hormonal imbalances.

What is the Difference Between Bio-identical Hormone Replacement Therapy (BHRT) and Hormone Replacement Therapy (HRT)?

Most people have heard of HRT as something that women take after menopause to improve mood and energy. HRT helps many women, but the concerns about breast cancer and heart problems have led many doctors to feel reluctant to prescribe it, or to only prescribe it to women for a few years to reduce the risks. I also see a lot of women who did not feel better with HRT and are looking for an alternative.

The reason why HRT can cause problems in the body is because, structurally, some of the hormones used are not exactly the same as the ones produced naturally by the body.

The benefits of bio-identical hormones are that they have fewer safety concerns than conventional HRT treatment, and can be compounded into tailor-made treatments, to suit each patient's unique set of symptoms and hormone levels. The main concerns over the use of conventional HRT are the proven increased risks of breast cancer, stroke and heart disease in patients on combined HRT with oestrogen and progesterone.[1] Bio-identical hormone therapy is a safer alternative, and can also be used where conventional treatment has failed or the side effects are too severe. Over two million women in the USA are using bio-identical hormone therapy presently and their use is on the increase in the UK and Europe. There are more and more doctors such as myself training in BHRT in the UK but at present it is only available privately in the UK.

Hormones Do Not Decline Because We Age – We Age Because Our Hormones Decline

Have you ever noticed how, after a certain age, women start to age more rapidly while men keep looking better and better? It's really not fair is it? But this is due to the rapid decline of female hormones.

Sue

Sue is a 50-year-old woman, and very typical of the women I see. She is still having menstrual periods but they are getting more irregular. Sue has two teenage children and still works. Although Sue looks well, she is constantly tired. She is starting to have hot flushes, and finds it hard to concentrate and have energy to exercise. She is snappy and irritable. Her sex drive has gone down massively. She finds it hard to cope with the stresses of everyday life. She cannot sleep well and as a result has no energy. She eats a good diet and is otherwise healthy.

This is a common case that I see on a regular basis. Sue's hormones are out of sync and it is causing her to feel out of balance and out of control of her energy, emotions and mood.

By testing and replacing low hormones and restoring the balance back in the body with the use of BHRT, I was able to help Sue get her energy and her life back.

By keeping hormone levels at optimal physiological levels it's possible to reduce osteoporosis, heart disease and strokes, and maintain brain function, memory, good sleep, energy, temperature regulation, weight-control, mood, skin tone and elasticity.

How balancing hormones can improve your health

- reduce fatigue
- reduce dry and wrinkled skin
- reduce mood swings and depression
- reduce symptoms of arthritis
- improve cholesterol levels
- improve sleep
- improve libido
- improve memory and concentration
- reduce hot flushes

HORMONE IMBALANCES

Before we look at how hormones can improve our health and energy, it's important to understand how they work in the body and what they do. I will go through each of the main hormones – oestrogen, progesterone, testosterone and dehydroepiandrosterone (DHEA) – in turn.

Firstly, it's important to note that all the major hormones are made from cholesterol as their starting building block. This is one of the reasons why I see women have a sudden rise in their cholesterol after the menopause, despite looking after their diet.

OESTROGEN

This is the hormone most people have heard about. Oestrogen is the female hormone that helps to regulate puberty, fertility and menopause and gives women their femininity, curves and softness. Approximately 300 different tissues are equipped with oestrogen receptors – such as the brain, liver, bones, the skin, blood vessels, breasts, urinary tract and uterus – and they rely on oestrogen to function effectively.

Symptoms relating to an imbalance in oestrogen

- vaginal dryness
- cystitis
- painful intercourse
- vaginal thrush
- urinary incontinence
- night sweats
- insomnia
- hot flushes
- depression and anxiety
- low energy
- memory loss
- mood swings
- headaches
- joint pains
- shortness of breath
- heart palpitations
- osteoporosis

Oestrogen is actually a group of three hormones: oestrone (E1), oestradiol (E2) and oestriol (E3).

Oestrone (E1) is the type of oestrogen most commonly found in increased amounts in post-menopausal women. Fifty per cent of oestrone is produced in the ovaries and the rest comes from hormones stored in the body fat. Oestrone can be broken down into a metabolite called 16-alpha-hydroxyoestrone, high levels of which have been observed in women with breast cancer. For this reason it is not commonly prescribed.

Oestradiol (E2) is the most potent type of oestrogen. It's responsible for the maturation of bones, development of the breasts, reproductive organs and female characteristics such as pubic hair and feminine curves. It's the primary oestrogen found in a woman's body during the reproductive years and is produced by the ovaries. Taking oestrodiol is very effective in reducing the symptoms of hot flushes during the menopause, low energy, vaginal and bladder irritation, preventing osteoporosis, increasing psychological well-being and reducing coronary artery disease.

Oestriol (E3) is the weakest of the three major oestrogens. Oestriol is made in large quantities during pregnancy and has protective properties against the production of cancerous cells. Oestriol is the oestrogen most beneficial to the vagina, cervix and vulva. Topical oestriol is very effective and the safest to use for vaginal dryness and can reduce vaginal irritation and cystitis. The lack of oestriol contributes to high numbers of urinary tract infections in older women.

The benefits of oestrogen

- body temperature regulation
- increased energy levels
- maintains bone density
- reduces the overall risk of heart disease
- decreases wrinkles
- increases libido
- enhances concentration
- lowers risk of colon cancer
- improves mood
- helps maintain memory
- maintains healthy muscles
- promotes restful sleep
- maintains artery elasticity
- increases blood flow
- maintains collagen levels in the skin

I often prescribe biest which is a combination of oestradiol and oestriol. It has the protective effects of oestriol while still providing the relief of symptoms such as hot flushes, low mood and energy, vaginal dryness and joint pains by oestradiol.

As I mention above, oestrone (E1) is not often prescribed in BHRT as it has the highest risk of breaking down into the substance called 16-alpha-hydroxyoestrone that is associated with breast cancer risk. But high levels of this substance are also associated with obesity, hypothyroidism, pesticide toxicity, high omega-5 fatty acid levels and high levels of inflammation. The body does naturally produce E1 and to reduce the chances of it being broken down into 16-alpha-hydroxyoestrone you can eat more broccoli, soya, flaxseeds, omega-3 fatty acids, rosemary and turmeric, as well as exercising and losing weight.

The Difference Between Oestradiol and Synthetic Oestrogen

The first thing it is important to know is that oestradiol in its bio-identical form is used in some conventional HRT. However, it is often put together with synthetic hormones in combination which means the full benefits are not seen. This is why some women do not experience benefit or have side effects from synthetic HRT prescribed by conventional doctors.

Premarin is a commonly used synthetic HRT. Premarin gets its name from the fact it is made from pregnant female horses' urine – **preg**nant-**mar**e's-ur**in**e. Premarin has been shown to stay in the body for up to 13 weeks, unlike oestradiol which, when substituted, is eliminated from the body within a few hours. This is due to the fact that the body's enzymes are designed to metabolise oestrogen and not synthetic oestrogen. Both oestradiol and premarin help maintain bone density, regulate body temperature and improve sleep patterns.

Differences in Oestradiol and Premarin

OESTRADIOL	PREMARIN
Increased HDL (good cholesterol) and lowered total cholesterol	Negatively altered blood lipids
Improved insulin sensitivity	Increased carbohydrate cravings
Inhibition of platelet stickiness	Increased triglycerides
Reduced accumulation of plaque on arteries	Increased risk of gallstones or cholestatic jaundice
Decreased blood pressure	Increased blood pressure
Reduced risk of heart disease	Elevated liver enzymes

PROGESTERONE

Progesterone is produced by the ovaries and adrenal glands in women, and in smaller amounts in the testes and adrenal glands in men. It's a vital hormone as it prepares the lining of the womb for implantation of a fertilised egg and helps maintain the embryo during pregnancy. Imbalances can be associated with endometriosis, fibroids, infertility, post-natal depression, having no periods and premenstrual tension.

Progesterone is important for brain function and is known as 'the happy hormone' because of its mood-enhancing and antidepressant effects. This may seem surprising to anyone taking the contraceptive pill with synthetic progesterone (known as progestogens) in it, as they are commonly known to make women feel depressed or cause mood swings.

Most women only associate oestrogen with female hormone function, but progesterone is just as vital during the menstruation years and is beneficial during the menopause. Progesterone levels decline faster than oestrogen levels during menopause. This imbalance between the two hormones can result in irregular or heavy periods, headaches and mood swings. Therefore

Symptoms relating to low progesterone

- mood swings
- heavy periods
- painful periods
- irritability
- low energy levels
- anxiety and depression
- osteoporosis
- insomnia
- decreased HDL levels (good cholesterol)

progesterone treatment is often preferred over oestrogen treatment as an initial remedy for menopausal symptoms.

In conventional medicine, it is a common misconception that progesterone is not needed in HRT if a woman has had a hysterectomy. This is not the case. Oestrogen and progesterone have a complementary effect and should always be prescribed together, even when a woman has had a hysterectomy. As already noted, progesterone is also needed for your mood and has other beneficial effects, other than keeping the lining of the womb thin.

The Differences Between Natural Progesterone and Progestogens

As with bio-identical oestrogen and synthetic oestrogens, there is a difference in the molecular structure of progesterone and provera, a commonly used synthetic progestogen. Whereas natural progesterone helps relieve depression and increase energy, synthetic progesterones do the opposite. Bio-identical progesterone also decreases blood pressure, reduces the risk of breast cancer, relieves the symptoms of PMT and improves fertility, while the progestins cause fluid retention, headaches, increase LDL (the 'bad' cholesterol), increase the risk of breast cancer and can cause breast tenderness and bloating, to name but a few effects.

TESTOSTERONE

In general, people think of testosterone as a male hormone and think it is not needed in women. This is incorrect. Women do produce testosterone, but in smaller amounts than men. The benefits of testosterone for women are increased libido, increased energy and motivation, increased muscle mass and strength, improved memory, mood and increased bone density.

Testosterone is often forgotten in females and is barely replaced in conventional HRT. The symptoms of low oestrogen such as hot flushes and vaginal dryness are hard to ignore, but the symptoms of low testosterone are often unrecognised yet can be as troublesome. Low levels of testosterone can cause fatigue, irritability, depression, aches and pains, thin skin, osteoporosis, weight loss, increased risk of heart attack and the loss of muscle.

Testosterone, like all hormones, needs to be dosed effectively or it can cause unwanted side effects like oily skin, acne, hair falling out or excessive body and facial hair, and can trigger aggression and anger.

Men and Testosterone Deficiency

Andropause, otherwise known as the 'male menopause', has attracted some press recently. Testosterone in men is produced in the testicles, and is at a peak in a man's mid-twenties. With age, the cells in the testicles begin to secrete less testosterone, and levels are also affected by stress, alcohol and medication. As well as reducing energy levels, causing depression and low libido, low levels of testosterone in men are associated with higher risks of death, heart attacks and strokes.[2]

DEHYDROEPIANDROSTERONE (DHEA)

DHEA is a steroid hormone and is produced by the adrenal glands, ovaries in women or testicles in men, and the brain. It is important for both men and women and increases energy levels, giving us that feeling of *joie de vivre*.

DHEA is a precursor to male and female sex hormones, which means it's a building block for the body to produce oestrogen and testosterone. It starts to decrease after the age of 30 and this drop correlates with the signs and symptoms of ageing. There has been much research into DHEA that shows it can be used to fight depression and fatigue, enhance feelings of well-being and increase strength. DHEA can also help with the symptoms of menopause, reducing body fat and improving libido.

Symptoms of low DHEA

- fatigue
- irritability
- depression
- weight gain
- low motivation

DHEA can be tested and replaced to help improve energy and your mood.

HORMONE CHANGES IN YOUNGER MEN AND WOMEN

There is a new trend in the hormones of young men. In their teens or early twenties they appear to be experiencing lower testosterone levels which cause low mood and low energy. Women are also experiencing changes in their hormone levels earlier and earlier, and are having longer peri-menopausal times, with hormone fluctuations sometimes starting 10 years before actual menopause and causing symptoms and changes in energy and mood. The evidence points to our exposure to chemicals in our food and environment.

I have first-hand experience of this. A few years ago I was feeling tired and lethargic, and struggling to lose weight despite a good diet and exercising. It wasn't until I went to a medical conference in the USA and had some specialised tests that I discovered I had high levels of oestrogen in my body, and that my testosterone was being converted to oestrogen. This explained why I was retaining weight, had low energy and had also been suffering with premenstrual tension for the first time in my life with severe pains around my ovaries. I also had another special-ised scan that showed the high levels of oestrogen had caused changes in my breasts that could lead to serious problems in the future if not corrected.

I stopped using anti-perspirant because one of the main ways to get rid of toxins in our body is through our sweat. I also had electro lymphatic drainage to stimulate my lymph glands around my breasts and armpits. This is because our lymphatic system is essential for clearing out waste and toxins from the body and is often impaired due to poor diet, lack of exercise and exposure to chemicals or electromagnetic radiation, such as from our mobile phones and Wi-Fi. I also started taking an aromatase inhibitor which stops the conversion of testosterone to oestrogen. These are commonly used to reduce oestrogen in breast cancer patients after surgery but I took a herbal version which worked really well for me.

I obviously wasn't pleased to have a hormone imbalance that could lead to serious problems if uncorrected, but I was grateful to have found the cause of my symptoms. This is why I really do understand how frustrating it can be to have disturbing symptoms, but be told by a medical professional that everything is fine.

Remember: *If you have symptoms, things are not fine. Your body is out of balance.* If you feel concerned speak to a doctor who has specialist knowledge in bio-identical hormones or hormone imbalances.

CASE STUDIES

Now that you understand how the different hormones work, let me give you some examples from my real-life patients on how they can help.

Premenstrual Tension – Cassie

Cassie, a 28-year-old woman, suffered with terrible premenstrual tension every month. It was so disabling she had to take time off work and felt very moody, tired and weak and often vomited because it was so severe. When her period came she had terrible pains and felt really unwell. She had a regular 28-day cycle and no other medical problems.

I started Cassie on progesterone cream to be used twice a day from days 18–28 of her menstrual cycle. After her first cycle using the progesterone cream she had fewer disabling symptoms, didn't vomit with her period, was able to go to work and didn't have to take any painkillers. After three months she didn't have any PMT symptoms at all – a life-changing experience for her.

Menopause – Linda

Linda, 54, went through menopause in her mid-40s. She took conventional HRT for a time but her GP stopped it two years ago as there's a family history of clots in the lungs and strokes, although she has no health problems of her own. She came to see me as she felt really tired and unfeminine. She also had zero libido and, with a younger husband, that side of her life was suffering. She had some hot flushes, her sleep was good and she was able to concentrate at work.

I checked Linda's blood tests and her natural levels of oestrogen, progesterone and testosterone were virtually nil. We started her on a lozenge with a good level of biest, progesterone and testosterone and the symptoms improved. We also did a urine oestrogen metabolism test which showed low levels of 16-alpha-hydroxyoesterone and high levels of 2-hydroxyoesterone so Linda had a low risk of breast cancer, clots and strokes.

Peri-menopause: Low Mood and Fatigue – Sandra

Sandra was 47 years old and had a low libido that was affecting her sex life. She felt very low in her mood and her energy, but she was still having regular periods.

I checked Sandra's blood tests and her FSH level, which is the hormone from the pituitary gland that signals to the ovaries to produce hormones, was normal, as was her progesterone and oestrogen levels. Her testosterone was virtually zero. This would be the cause of her low libido, her low mood and tiredness. I prescribed a testosterone cream to be used once a day every day throughout her cycle for her to use on the inside of her arms to be absorbed through the skin, and also in her genital area to stimulate her libido and increase sensitivity. After five weeks Sandra noticed an improvement in her energy, mood and sex drive, and after three months, her clitoral and vaginal sensitivity returned and she felt back to her usual self again.

Hormonal Migraines – Kelly

Kelly, 42, was having regular periods, but experiencing migraines mid-cycle and just before her period started. She also felt low in her mood, ate a lot and was overweight. She felt a bit anxious too.

Her FSH level was normal, showing she was not in menopause. Her testosterone levels, DHEA and progesterone were all normal. Her oestrogen was more than 10 times higher than her progesterone levels. High oestrogen levels in comparison to progesterone levels can cause headaches. In some women, low oestrogen levels can also cause headaches. I started Kelly on progesterone cream twice a day from days 12–28 of her cycle, and after six weeks her headaches were much improved. However, she was still having headaches during her periods. She used the cream from days 12–28 and days one to five of her period, and after three months the headaches were still there, but much improved, and they did not stop her from being active.

Fibroids – Holly

Holly, 35, had a history of heavy periods and fibroids. Her fibroids had grown in the last two years and her periods were heavier with flooding and clots. It affected her life because she felt worried to go out during her period in case she had an accident. Because of the heavy bleeding this was leading to anaemia. She had tried a mirena coil to reduce the bleeding but couldn't tolerate it due to the size of the fibroids in her womb. She had seen a gynaecologist who recommended a hysterectomy. However, Holly didn't want to completely eliminate her chances of having a baby.

I discussed using high-dose progesterone treatment to help alleviate Holly's symptoms. Her blood tests showed a high oestradiol level and a low progesterone level. The high levels of oestrogen were not being balanced by progesterone so this contributed to the increase in bleeding and the growth of the fibroids. After three months of using progesterone as a lozenge throughout her cycle – a lower amount from days 1–14 of the cycle and a higher dose from days 15–28 – the blood flow was much lower and her periods were regular. A repeated ultrasound showed that the fibroids had reduced in size and the lining of her womb was of a normal thickness. She was taking iron and, because the bleeding was less, her anaemia had resolved.

Hot Flushes and Night Sweats – Carole

When Carole came to me she was 54 and had had her last period one year ago. She had tried conventional HRT but it hadn't helped at all. Her main problem was that she had hot flushes every half an hour and night sweats that affected her sleep every night. Her mood was okay, she was getting headaches but she felt tired all the time and the flushes were embarrassing when she went out and about. Her libido was low too.

Carole's FSH levels were high. Her oestradiol levels were low, as were her testosterone and progesterone levels. This indicated she was in menopause. I started her on a cream containing biest, progesterone and testosterone to be used twice a day every day. After four weeks her hot flushes had virtually disappeared, except for a few at night. Her sleep was better but she still had headaches, but her energy level improved. We increased the dose after eight weeks and then her night sweats disappeared with the headaches and her energy was back to normal.

Urinary Incontinence – Brenda

Brenda, 56, had not had a period for two years. She had really severe vaginal dryness and couldn't have sex due to the discomfort. To make matters worse, she also had urinary incontinence every day meaning she had to wear a panty liner all the time. Her libido was low and her mood flat.

Brenda had a high FSH level showing she was in menopause, and had undetectable levels of oestradiol, progesterone and testosterone. I started her on a cream containing a mixture of oestradiol, progesterone and testosterone to be used every day for two weeks, and also started her on Vagifem, which are vaginal pessaries of bio-identical oestrogen, to help improve the vaginal tissues, which are used every day for two weeks and then three times a week. After three months her vaginal tissues were improved, she was having less urinary incontinence and she was able to have sexual intercourse with her husband. Her mood and libido had also improved.

Pain and Arthritis – Debbie

At 52, Debbie's last period was four years ago. She had painful joints, hips and back. She was diagnosed with severe osteoarthritis and a carpal tunnel syndrome. She was also having hot flushes, fatigue and insomnia.

Her FSH levels were high, her oestradiol levels were low, as were her testosterone and progesterone levels. We tested her vitamin D levels, which were low and her DHEA was low. Her bone density tests showed mild osteoporosis. I started her on a lozenge with biest, progesterone, testosterone and DHEA twice a day, and vitamin D for three months. After four weeks, Linda had fewer joint pains and her carpal tunnel syndrome had improved so she was taking fewer painkillers. She had more energy, felt more alert and her hot flushes were lessened.

Low Energy and Tiredness – Sabrina

Sabrina is a 36-year-old woman with regular but heavy periods and tiredness. Her energy was low despite eating well. She exercised but only once a week as she had a busy job and a hectic social life. Her sex drive and mood were good. She had some PMT symptoms but they weren't too severe.

Sabrina had normal female hormonal levels when tested. Her DHEA levels were low. DHEA can convert into testosterone which will also help energy. We substituted the DHEA and after three months her energy levels were much better.

Low Energy and Libido in a Man – Ryan

Ryan is a 54-year-old man who is becoming increasingly tired and putting on weight around his middle. He also is no longer able to maintain an erection and his libido has gone down. He is married and his relationship is suffering due to this. He is otherwise fit and well and has a great diet and exercises regularly.

I tested Ryan's hormones and his DHEA was normal but his testosterone was at the bottom range of normal. We replaced his testosterone with a cream and he felt better within three months and was able to get his sex drive back. He also lost seven pounds.

I hope that you can see that problems due to hormone imbalances can be successfully treated with the right prescription of hormones, tailored to each individual and their needs, as well as having added health benefits. Having distressing symptoms of the menopause, or experiencing erratic, painful periods, is not something that has to be endured. Balancing your hormones can also help slow down the ageing process and improve your mood and energy.

CONCLUSION

Well done and thank you for making it to the end of the book! If you've completed the energy cleanse plan then I know you'll have come out the other side feeling better than ever. I'm proud of you, and you should be too – proud of the commitment you've made to take responsibility for your well-being.

This is just the beginning. You now need to sustain your wonderful work in order to keep feeling this good. It won't always be easy when you're busy and life certainly has a tendency to get in the way. The good news is you've built a foundation upon which new habits can form. Consistency is now key to make them part of your daily routine. Good habits will help you to make healthy choices long term and keep you feeling well and full of vitality. Going forward, whenever you need to remind yourself of the principles in this book and stay on track, I'd like you to revisit this guidance:

THE RULES TO KEEP TIREDNESS AWAY AND FEEL FULL OF VITALITY FOR LIFE

1. SMALL CHANGES MAKE A BIG DIFFERENCE
As the saying goes, Rome wasn't built in a day. There's a lot of information in this book and much of it may have been new to you. I don't want you to do everything at once and become overwhelmed.

As I said at the beginning, I'm just like you. Despite being an expert in this area I still can't resist every bar of chocolate or having a takeaway now and then, and I certainly skive off the gym from time to time. It's challenging to make changes when they feel very different to how we're hard-wired to behave (instant gratification being one) and we're constantly being given contradictory messages from our media and main food providers, the supermarkets.

It can seem overwhelming when you look at yourself and think about going from where you are today to being superhealthy and fit, so set yourself small and obtainable goals every week instead of looking at the mountain you have to climb.

For example, try not to think about going from your current level of fitness to running a marathon. Instead, think about going from where you are today to doing a walk 10 minutes a day for a week, then a brisk walk 20 minutes the week after and 30 minutes the week after that with intermittent jogging and so on. Break your goals into small steps to make them more tangible and realistic. Every goal is possible, just start the journey with a single step.

2. GIVE IT TIME

It will take time to get your health and vitality back on track. You're a work in progress. We all are. If you decided tomorrow to go from just chilling out on your sofa watching television and eating cake to becoming a full-time, vegan, yoga-loving meditator, then you're just setting yourself up to fail. New habits take time to form and so making small, obtainable changes (as above) and sticking to them is the key to success. Choose one or two changes a week and be consistent, and once it comes easily to you then add in something else. Be kind with yourself and exercise patience with your body and mind. You'll get there.

3. GET IN TUNE WITH YOUR BODY

It's important to become in tune with your body and learn to recognise the messages it gives you. When I'm run-down I often crave oranges, which are full of vitamin C, or ginger, which has natural anti-inflammatory properties. Other times I may crave a rich vegetable soup full of nutrients. When I'm tired I often crave beetroot, which can help to increase blood count levels and therefore improves energy. When I'm aching it's my body's sign to stretch and relax. Over the years I've learned to become the expert on me. Long before I was diagnosed with high oestrogen in my body, I already knew I had a female disorder of some sort due to experiencing various symptoms such as lower pains in my pelvis and new post-menstrual tension. I get headaches when I'm not sleeping enough or when I'm dehydrated. I understand how my body works, and while I know I have the advantage of being a doctor trained in integrative medicine, I believe anyone can learn to listen to what their body is telling them and understand themselves better.

It takes time, meditation, being really honest with yourself and noticing patterns that happen within your body. A useful method is to keep a mood and food diary as mentioned in chapter 8 (see page 86). Keep a record of the foods you eat, and how you feel emotionally and physically. For example, if after eating chocolate cake you feel tired and have a hollow feeling in your stomach then you know that the cake isn't reacting well in your body.

4. NO ONE SHOULD CARE MORE ABOUT YOU THAN YOU DO YOURSELF

This is the truth. Your doctor, friends and family can all help you along the way, but no one should care more for you than you do. Your health is your number one priority. This may be contrary to how you've been living, possibly putting others before yourself, but you picked up this book for a reason – because you know your health is not as good as it should be, or you don't feel as good as you think you can.

We're all guilty of thinking that serious illness won't happen to us, that it's something that happens to someone else and we become complacent. Unfortunately, due to the nature of my work, I know this isn't true and have seen first-hand, on more occasions than I wish to remember, how devastating and painful this can be. When you or a loved one falls ill, it changes everything. Self-care and nurturing can prevent this from happening, so there's no excuse not to take control, step up and take responsibility and make the changes *now* before it's too late.

5. WORK ON THE 70/30 RULE

If you are 'good' and eat well, exercise and manage your stress for 70 per cent of the time then your 'well-being bank balance' will stay in the black. This is equivalent to looking after yourself for five days a week so that for the other two days you can have a takeaway, some wine, cake or chocolates. That doesn't sound too bad, does it? It's about balance, and looking after your health but not making it into a chore. I genuinely believe if you look after your health extremely well 70 per cent of the time then it doesn't matter what you do for the remainder, within reason, so you can let your hair down and relax.

6. EXERCISE

Keeping your body moving is the best way to keep feeling full of vitality, energy and life. The World Health Organization recommends doing half an hour of exercise, five days a week. This is a good start. Keep moving, even if it's only walking. It's beneficial to try and get a balance between cardiovascular exercise and core exercises that work on posture and balance, such as yoga and Pilates. Even going for a walk contributes to your fitness and has the added bonus of getting out in the fresh air.

7. STRESS MANAGEMENT

Spend time every day relaxing and de-stressing, even if it's only for 10 minutes a day. Remember to keep up with your relaxation and breathing exercises. Spending time doing anything you enjoy is always beneficial and not self-indulgent. So make time to read a book, treat yourself to a massage, have a relaxing bath or go dancing! Remember that when you're happy and free from stress, you're functioning optimally to give your best to others so don't ever feel guilty about it.

8. SUPPLEMENTS

As standard, take a good food-based multivitamin supplement a day. Also take omega-3 fish oils, a probiotic and vitamin D supplements. These are just the basics. For someone who is fit and healthy this should be more than adequate. If you have further health problems then you may need extra supplementation. For example, if you have low mood you may benefit from extra B vitamins. Some people will benefit from taking an extra antioxidant if their immune system is low. If you need any further advice on supplements then contact a health-care professional like myself who is trained in integrative medicine, functional medicine or is a naturopath, who will understand the benefits of supplementation and what your needs may be. Remember that your conventional GP or doctor plays an important and essential role in treating illness and disease, but has not necessarily been trained to understand the benefits of supplements and how they work so they're not always the best people to speak to about this topic.

9. BE KIND TO YOURSELF

From time to time we all have periods where we overindulge. Remember this is just temporary, don't punish yourself and just start again. For example, if you're going away on holiday, or it's Christmas or your birthday you should enjoy it. Be comfortable knowing that you now have the tools to set yourself back on track, time and again. There will also be times where you feel run-down and unwell. When this happens it's important to rest and take extra supplements of elderberry, zinc, vitamin C and beta glucans to boost your immunity. At any time you can just go back to a week of 'eating clean' if you feel your energy or health need a boost, or do the three-week plan to really give yourself a deeper cleanse.

10. YOUR HEALTH IS A COMBINATION OF FOUR KEY AREAS

In my experience, you can't achieve total health unless you look at a combination of exercise, nutrition, managing stress and cutting out vices. For example, you can eat really healthily, go to the gym five times a week and do yoga for your stress, but if you drink alcohol like a fish or smoke you simply can't achieve total health. If you don't smoke or drink, eat well, manage stress but do no exercise you also can't achieve optimum health. Likewise, if you're a gym bunny and not stressed, don't smoke or drink but live on junk food you won't be fully healthy either. All four of these areas need to be met to achieve total health. Remember: sugar is a vice that's as bad as smoking or excessive alcohol consumption and needs to be managed and restricted in the same way.

11. OTHER IMBALANCES

There can be other imbalances that need correcting in the body, especially if after following the three-week energy cleanse you don't feel 100 per cent well. For example, there could be an adrenal, chemical or hormonal imbalance. This normally requires further investigation and a more in-depth, personal consultation. If this is something you're worried about then please get in touch with a holistic health-care professional. The most important thing when choosing a health-care professional is that you feel they understand you and you connect with them and feel they'll treat your condition in the way you feel is appropriate, with the right balance of the conventional medical and a more natural approach.

12. DON'T FORGET HOW YOU FELT BEFORE

Remember how you felt before embarking on this programme, or the time when your health was at its worst? Sometimes when we feel good or even just okay we forget what it was like before and it becomes harder to motivate ourselves to make those key life-style changes. If you recall the time you felt your worst and how different your lifestyle was at that time it will keep you motivated to make or continue positive changes in your life. Acknowledge this and recommit.

13. REMEMBER WHY THIS IS IMPORTANT TO YOU

What do you want *out of your life?* What goals do you want to achieve? Could it be to get a better job, meet a partner, travel more, see your children or grandchildren grow up and have families themselves? Whatever your personal hopes and dreams, you have to be fit and well to make them happen and to see and experience everything you wish for.

How do you want to feel? Is it happy, full of energy, successful, loving and loved, or have a sense of pride in yourself? Spend time every day visualising this and really feel the emotions. Hang on to this feeling to keep you motivated to reach your goals. A common way this is used in sports teams is to use visualisation to improve scoring. Research has shown that when one group practises their shooting only, while another group doesn't do any physical practice but visualises themselves shooting and scoring perfectly every time, the group that had the best outcomes when they all go back to training was the group who visualised but did not practise. This shows how powerful the mind is in guiding us to our goals.

Who do you want to be to your family and loved ones? Someone they can respect, someone who teaches them good habits and sets a fantastic and inspirational example? You can be all these things and more, if you're willing to put some work in. Use your answers to these questions to keep you inspired to reach your goals and take the steps to make them happen.

14. THINK ABOUT WHAT DRAINS YOUR ENERGY

In addition to eating well, exercising and taking supplements, you may need to consider other factors as there may be other influences that drain your energy. For example, your body may need extra help dealing with pollution, or you could be reacting to the chemicals you use in your home, body products or on your clothes. It's important to try to minimise these wherever possible. Remember in chapter 7 we discussed how chemicals in your body are a major predictor of future health, obesity and illness? So this really does matter. Switch to chemical-free beauty and household products as much as possible. There are fantastic skincare, body products and make-up on the market now that are chemical-free. They may be slightly pricey but it's worth the investment to improve your overall health.

Next, consider the psychological and emotional energy drainers in your life. These can be in the form of people who are negative and bring you down, your job, or focusing on what you lack in life rather than what you have. When you are in a difficult situation it's a major drain on your natural energy. Try to take small steps to resolve the problems you're facing by either resolving each one or, if this is not possible, reframing them in a different way. For example, if you don't like your job, remind yourself it pays for you to do fun things at the weekend and take lovely holidays. If there's someone draining in your life try to take a step away from them, or minimise your time with them, but if it's not entirely possible, feel thankful that they've taught you patience and tolerance and are making you a better person.

15. PUT YOURSELF FIRST

You may have commitments to your family, your job and your friends, but from time to time you need to schedule regular time for you. If you're not on top form, then you won't have enough energy and spirit to do everything you need to do well. I never feel guilty about scheduling in time for myself. I regularly give myself time off to watch television or a film, go out to see friends or take a long walk. I know that when I feel good and relaxed, I can give my best to my friends, patients and work. Most importantly, I'm giving my best to myself and being the best version of 'me' I can be. It's not selfish; it's the greatest gift you can give to yourself and those you love.

16. CUT OUT THE BAD STUFF

In my own health, I've found that until I've massively reduced the 'bad stuff', the 'good stuff' doesn't get a chance to show its full effect. Let me give you my example. I've been juicing for years so I've been getting more than my 'five a day' and have also been taking numerous supplements. However, initially I wasn't feeling the benefit. It can be easy to then say the 'good stuff' isn't working. It wasn't until I cut out the 'bad stuff' that I felt differently. I cut out sugar and reduced my wheat and dairy and felt so much better. That's just the way life is. If you can stick to the 70/30 rule and make sure you have four to five 'eating clean' days a week, you *will* see the difference.

17. YOU ARE STILL 'YOU' EVEN THOUGH YOU'RE HEALTHY

So much of our identity is closely linked to how we socialise. It took me a long time to get my head around the fact I could still be fun and healthy. You may feel like you won't be the same person without five alcoholic drinks on a night out, or your friends will think you're boring if you stop smoking or start eating healthier and pass on the chips. You are still you, but you'll be the best version of yourself. Healthy doesn't have to equal boring. In fact, you'll have so much energy you will be the most fun person in the room, with or without an alcoholic drink.

18. WHAT IS THE ONE THING YOU'RE RESISTING THE MOST?

I once heard a colleague say that he often tells his patients they need to think about whatever it is they're resisting in their health as, generally, that's what will bring about the greatest benefit to their health and well-being. This completely resonated with me when I heard it because it's so true.

Think about it. What are you resisting doing the most for your health, even though you know it's good for you?

For me, it would be exercise and waking up earlier. My diet is good and I take supplements and I manage my stress well, but I often make excuses to avoid the gym and prefer to have my morning lie-in. I like to tell myself that because I eat well and take my supplements I don't have to exercise as much. However, I know that this isn't really true (see point 10 page 224). I know deep down that it's the one thing that will make the biggest difference to my health, but I tell myself I don't have the time to do it because I know how much hard work it will be to get going, and how long it would take to build up my fitness!

So, it's important to be really honest with yourself about what you're avoiding and why. If you want to improve your energy and achieve true health and well-being then you have to do the thing you want to do the least. What are YOU resisting? It is the one thing that will bring you the most benefit. This one answer can be applied to almost any aspect of your life and will cause major transformations. If you take only one thing from this book, then this is it.

19. DO THE THREE-WEEK ENERGY CLEANSE ON A REGULAR BASIS

Whenever you feel run-down or lethargic, or life's excesses have got in the way, do the three-week cleanse to reset your metabolism and energy. I would recommend doing the plan at least once every six months. If you are feeling run-down or unwell and feel like you need a little boost, do a week of 'eating clean' which is week one of the three-week plan.

20. GET SUPPORT

It's incredibly hard to stay on track and be healthy if you don't have any support. Curiously it's often the people closest to us who don't support us. It isn't that they don't care, it's often that they're just resistant to change and worry that if you change you won't be the same person or feel the same about them. If you can't find support at home, make friends who can help you in your new healthy quest or join an online group like the ones I run for my clients. This is why people who attend slimming groups are often more successful than when they try to go it alone. Find at least one person to support you and keep one another motivated by celebrating your wins and consoling each other if you fall off the wagon. If you can't meet in person, then calls and texts work well too. Knowing that someone is always there for you will help strengthen your resolve to succeed and ensure you get better results.

21. CONSISTENCY IS KEY

I've been abroad for detox retreats, spent a lot of money, eaten amazingly well and exercised like a demon, and then come home and gone back to my usual lifestyle. I realised it was pointless being incredibly healthy and pious for one week, and then spending the other 51 weeks eating crisps. There are no health benefits to that. Consistency is key. Try and make small changes *every day* that benefit your health.

22. HAVE A MINIMUM TWO TO THREE 'CLEAN EATING' DAYS A WEEK

The best way to maintain your health and wellness is to have two or three 'clean eating' days a week although four to five days is preferable if you are trying to really improve your health. This will give your body the time to heal from any strain put on it from eating products such as dairy, wheat or processed foods and drinks. The constant assault of consuming these products daily without a rest means that the body never has a chance to recover and this can lead to inflammation and eventually disease in the body. Eating clean for several days, preferably in a row, gives the body a chance to regenerate and rest.

23. LEARN TO COOK AND BUY LOCAL PRODUCE

It's hard to know what's in food when you buy it pre-prepared. 'Food fraud' is a real problem where we can't be sure what meat is in our pre-prepared meals, what sort of fish is inside the batter, and there have even been claims that some shop-bought fruit juices, such as orange and apple, are substituted with sugary syrup. Other foods that are prone to food fraud are olive oil, coffee, honey and saffron. These foods may not be as pure as they say on the label. The best thing to do, if possible, is to buy from a local producer who you can question about what is in the products you're buying.

Learn to make healthy and nutritious versions of your favourite meals. This way you can always have enjoyable and delicious meals and not feel guilty or have to worry about what you may be putting in your body.

24. WHEN ALL ELSE FAILS, DUST YOURSELF OFF AND START AGAIN

No one is perfect and we're often too hard on ourselves. It's hard in modern life to stick to health plans when they don't come naturally to you. Remind yourself that *we're all just doing the best we can with what we have at this moment in time*. Instead of beating yourself up, just remember that we're all human and fall off the wagon from time to time. Simply dust yourself off and start again. If you've slipped up recently or had a period of excess then just choose a week of eating clean or start the three-week cleanse again.

I hope this book has helped you to see that obtaining good health and well-being is easier than perhaps you thought it could be, and that there are trained health professionals who are committed to helping you have the best wellness you can and guide you along this path.

I wish you the very best in health and happiness. May you always have the energy you deserve to enjoy your life!

REFERENCES

Chapter 1
1. Roberts, Michelle. 'UK "fares badly in European health league table"' http://www.bbc.co.uk/news/health-21654536
2. Ornish, Dean Dr. *The Spectrum: A Scientifically Proven Program to Feel Better, Live Longer, Lose Weight and Gain Health* (New York: Ballantine Books, 2007)
3. Preece, Rob. 'Did this grandfather, 78, really beat "incurable" cancer by just changing his diet?' September 2012, Mail Online, http://www.dailymail.co.uk/health/article-2204080/Grandfather-incurable-cancer-given-clear-swapping-red-meat-dairy-products-10-fruit-veg-day.html
4. http://www.nobelprize.org/nobel_prizes/medicine/laureates/2009/press.html
5. With thanks to Dr Mark Atkinson for permission to use his questionnaire: www.drmarkatkinson.com

Chapter 2
1. NHS Choices online – anaemia, iron deficiency, http://www.nhs.uk/conditions/Anaemia-iron-deficiency-/Pages/Introduction.aspx
2. NHS Choices online – anaemia, vitamin B12 or folate, http://www.nhs.uk/conditions/anaemia-vitamin-b12-and-folate-deficiency/Pages/Introduction.aspx
3. Patient.co.uk – pernicious anaemia and B12 deficiency, http://www.patient.co.uk/doctor/pernicious-anaemia-and-b12-deficiency
4. NHS Choices – Live Well. 10 Medical Reasons for Feeling Tired, http://www.nhs.uk/Livewell/tiredness-and-fatigue/Pages/medical-causes-of-tiredness.aspx
5. NHS Choices online – Fibromyalgia, http://www.nhs.uk/Conditions/Fibromyalgia/Pages/Introduction.aspx
6. NHS Choices online – Chronic Fatigue Syndrome, http://www.nhs.uk/Conditions/Chronic-Fatigue-Syndrome/pages/introduction.aspx

Chapter 3

1. Shrivastava, A, Tiwari, M, Sinha, RA, et al. 'Molecular iodine induces caspase-independent apoptosis in human breast carcinoma cells involving the mitochondria-mediated pathway.' *Journal of Biological Chemistry*, 2006 Jul 14; 281(28): 19762–71.

2. Eskin, BA, Grotkowski, CE, Connolly, CP, Ghent, WR. 'Different tissue responses for iodine and iodide in rat thyroid and mammary glands.' *Biological Trace Element Research*, 1995 Jul; 49(1): 9–19.

3. Fazio, S, Palmieri, EA, Lombardi, G, Biondi, B. 'Effects of thyroid hormone on the cardiovascular system.' *Recent Progress in Hormone Research*, 2004; 59: 31–50.

4. Abnet, CC, Fan, JH, Kamangar, F, et al. 'Self-reported goiter is associated with a significantly increased risk of gastric noncardia adenocarcinoma in a large population-based Chinese cohort.' *International Journal of Cancer*, 2006 Sep 15; 119(6): 1508–10.

5. Golkowski, F, Szybinski, Z, Rachtan, J, et al. 'Iodine prophylaxis – the protective factor against stomach cancer in iodine deficient areas.' *European Journal of Nutrition* 2007 Aug; 46(5): 251–6.

Chapter 4

1. Atkinson, Mark Dr. *The Mind–Body Bible*, (London: Piatkus, 2007)
2. www.adrenalfatigue.org
3. Yang, G, et al. 'Treatment of Allergic Rhinitis with Probiotics: An Alternative Approach.' *North American Journal of Medical Science.* 2013 Aug; 5(8): 465–468
4. Daniells, S. 'Kefir ingredients could help food allergies.' October 2006, NUTRA ingredients.com, http://www.nutraingredients.com/Research/Kefir-ingredients-could-help-food-allergies

Chapter 5

1. Marsden, Kathryn. *Good Gut Bugs*, (London: Piatkus, 2010)
2. Kang, E, et al. 'The Effect of Probiotics on Prevention of Common Cold: A Meta-Analysis of Randomized Controlled Trial Studies.' *Korean Journal of Family Medicine.* 2013; 34(1): 2–10

Chapter 6

1. Gillespie, David. *Sweet Poison: Why Sugar Makes Us Fat* (London: Penguin, 2013)

2. Scarborough, P. et al. 'The economic burden of ill health due to diet, physical inactivity, smoking, alcohol and obesity in the UK: an update to 2006-07 NHS costs.' *Journal of Public Health (Oxf)*. 2011 Dec; 33(4): 52735. doi: 10.1093/pubmed/fdr033. Epub 2011

3. Stanhope, KL. 'Role of fructose-containing sugars in the epidemics of obesity and metabolic syndrome.' *Annual Review of Medicine*, 2012; 63: 32943. doi: 10.1146/annurev-med-042010-113026. Epub 2011 http://www.ncbi.nlm.nih.gov/pubmed/22034869

4. Lustig, Robert Dr. *Fat Chance: The Bitter Truth About Sugar*, (London: Fourth Estate, 2013)

5. Burdakov, et al. 'Activation of central orexin/hypocretin neurons by dietary amino-acids', *Neuron*, 2011.

6. Yudkin, John. *Pure, White and Deadly: How Sugar is Killing Us and What We Can Do to Stop It*, (London: Penguin, 2012)

7. Keys, Ancel. The Seven Countries Study, http://www.epi.umn.edu/cvdepi/study.asp?id=12

8. Malhotra, Aseem. 'Saturated fat is not the major issue.' *British Medical Journal*, 2013; 347 doi: http://dx.doi.org/10.1136/bmj.f6340 (Published 22 October 2013)

9. Lê, KA, et al. 'Fructose overconsumption causes dyslipidemia and ectopic lipid deposition in healthy subjects with and without a family history of type 2 diabetes.' *American Journal of Clinical Nutrition*. 2009 Jun; 89(6):1760-5. doi: 10.3945/ajcn.2008.27336. Epub 2009 Apr 29. http://www.ncbi.nlm.nih.gov/pubmed/19403641

10. Williams, Rhiannon, et. al. 'Adaptive sugar sensors in hypothalamic feeding circuits.' *Proceedings of the National Academy of Sciences of the United States of America*. http://www.pnas.org/content/105/33/11975.full

11. Nettleton, JA, et al. 'Diet soda intake and risk of incident metabolic syndrome and type 2 diabetes in the multi-ethnic study of atherosclerosis (MESA).' *American Diabetes Association Diabetic Care Journal*, http://care.diabetesjournals.org/content/32/4/688

12. Lenoir, H, et al, 'Intense sweetness surpasses cocaine reward.' *PLOS One*, 2007. http://www.ncbi.nlm.nih.gov/pubmed/17668074

Chapter 7

1. Scientific Committee in Food, 2000. Opinion of the SCF on the Risk Assessment of dioxins and dioxin-like PCBs in Food. European Commission, Health Cons Prot Dir Gen, Bruxelles.

2. Ha, MH, et al. 'Association between serum concentrations of persistent organic pollutants and self-reported cardiovascular disease prevalence: results from the National Health and Nutrition Examination Survey 1999–2002.' *Environmental Health Perspectives*, Aug 2007; 115(8): 1204–9

3. Ha MH, et al. 'Association between serum concentrations of persistent organic pollutants and prevalence of newly diagnosed hypertension: results from the National Health and Nutrition Examination Survey 1999–2002.' *Journal of Human Hypertension*, Apr 2009, 23(4): 274–86

4. Smink, A, et al. 'Exposure to hexachlorobenzene during pregnancy increases the risk of overweight in children aged 6 years' *Acta Paediatrica*, 2008; 97, 1465-1469

5. Schell, LM, et al. 'Pollution and human biology.' Annals of Human Biology, 2010, June; 37(3):347-66

6. Lee, DH, et al. 'A strong dose-response relation between serum concentrations of persistent organic pollutants and diabetes'. Results from the National Health and Examination Survey 1999–2002. *Diabetes Care*, 2006

7. Laboratory tests for POPs:
   Metametrix – www.metametrix.com
   Pacific Toxicology – www.pactox.com
   NMS reference labs – www.nmslab.com
   Rocky Mountain Analytical – www.rmalab.com

8. Lee, DH, et al. 'Serum GGT predicts non-fatal myocardial infarction and fatal coronary heart disease among 28,838 middle-aged men and women.' *European Heart Journal*, 2006; 27:2170-6

9. Lee, DH, et al, 'GGT and diabetes – a four-year follow-up study.' *Diabetologia*. Mar 2003; 46(3):359-64

10. Lee, DH, et al. 'Can persistent organic pollutants explain the association between serum GGT and type 2 diabetes?' *Diabetologia*, 2008 March; 51(3): 402-7

11. Lu C, et al. 'Dietary intake and its contribution to longitudinal organophosphorus pesticide exposure in urban/suburban children.' *Environmental Health Perspectives*, Apr 2008; 116(4) 537–42

Chapter 8

1. Oyebode, O, Gordon-Dseagu, V, Walker, A, Mindell, JS. 'Fruit and vegetable consumption and all-cause, cancer and CVD mortality: analysis of Health Survey for England data.' *Journal of Epidemiology*

and Community Health. Published online March 2014, http://
jech.bmj.com/content/early/2014/03/03/jech-2013-203500.
abstract?sid=37308e66-df0a-4277-89c5-8917a1d18dab

2. 'Britons spend more money on chocolate than any other country in
   Europe, *Daily Telegraph*, 8 October 2009. http://www.telegraph.
   co.uk/finance/newsbysector/retailandconsumer/6272067/Britons-
   spend-more-on-chocolate-than-any-country-in-Europe.html

3. 'Takeaway UK: Average Brit is now spending £1,320 a year on fast
   food buying 12 meals every month.' Mail Online, 5 April 2013.
   http://www.dailymail.co.uk/news/article-2303861/Takeaway-UK-
   Average-Brit-spending-1-320-year-fastfood-buying-12-meals-month.
   html#ixzz2zZK8HWjN

4. Barnouin K, Freedman R. *Skinny Bitch*, (Philadelphia: Running Press,
   2005)

5. Bowden, Jonny. *The Healthiest Meals on Earth*, (London: Fair Winds
   Press, 2008)

6. Bell, JG, et al. 'Dioxin and dioxin-like polychlorinated biphenyls
   (PCBs) in Scottish farmed salmon (Salmo salar): effects of replacement
   of dietary marine fish oil with vegetable oils'. *Aquaculture*, Volume 243,
   Issues 1–4, January 2005, 305–314

7. http://preventdisease.com/news/12/032012_Why-80-Percent-of-
   People-Worldwide-Will-Soon-Stop-Eating-Wheat.shtml

8. Shepherd, SJ, et al. 'Dietary triggers of abdominal symptoms in
   patients with irritable bowel syndrome: randomized placebo-controlled
   evidence.' *Clinical Gastroenterology and Hepatology*, Jul 2008; 6(7):
   765–71

9. *Food, Inc.* documentary 2009. Directed by Robert Kenner.

10. www.ewg.org/foodnews/summary.php

11. Smith-Spangler, C, et al. 'Are organic foods safer or healthier than
    conventional alternatives?: a systematic review.' *Annals of Internal
    Medicine*, Sep 2012, Volume 157, Number 5

12. Ebbeling Cara, 'Effects of dietary composition on energy expenditure
    during weight-loss maintenance.' *Journal of the American Medical Asso-
    ciation*, 2012

13. Cheng, B, et al. 'Coffee components inhibit amyloid formation of
    human islet amyloid polypeptide in vitro: possible link between coffee
    consumption and diabetes mellitus.' *Journal of Agricultural & Food
    Chemistry*, Dec 2011, 59(24): 13147–55

14. Ponte, M, et al. 'Coffee drinking associated with lower risk for alcohol-related liver disease.' *Archives of Internal Medicine*, 2006; 166: 1190–1195

15. Chuanhai, Cao, et al. 'High blood caffeine levels in MCI linked to lack of progression to dementia.' *Journal of Alzheimer's Disease*, 29 (2012) 1–14

16. Lucas, M, et al. 'Coffee, caffeine, and the risk of completed suicide: results from three prospective cohorts of American adults.' *World Journal of Biological Psychiatry*, July 2013

17. Costill, DL, et al. 'Effects of caffeine ingestion on metabolism and exercise performance.' *Medicine and Science in Sports*, 1978, 10(3): 155–158

18. Davy, BM, et al. 'Water consumption reduces energy intake at a breakfast meal in obese older adults.' *Journal of the American Dietetic Association*, Volume 108, Issue 7, July 2008, 1236–1239

CHAPTER 9

1. Chalder, T, et al. 'Development of a Fatigue Scale', *Journal of Psychosomatic Research*, Volume 37, No 2, 1993, 147–153

2. Vallejo, F, et al. 'Phenolic compound contents in edible parts of broccoli inflorescences after domestic cooking.' *Journal of the Science of Food and Agriculture*, Nov 2003, Volume 83, Issue 14, pages 1511–1516

3. *Healthy Eating: A Guide to the New Nutrition*, a Harvard Medical School Special Report

4. Brown, Jeff and Fenske, Mark. *The Winner's Brain: 8 Strategies Great Minds Use to Achieve Success*, (Cambridge, Mass: Da Capo Press, 2010)

CHAPTER 10

1. Cohen, S, et al. 'Sleep habits and susceptibility to the common cold.' *Archives of Internal Medicine*, 2009; 169(1): 62–67

2. Axelsson, J, et al. 'Beauty sleep: experimental study on the perceived health and attractiveness of sleep deprived people.' *British Medical Journal*, 2010; 341:c6614

3. Kripke DF, Langer RD, Kline LE. 'Hypnotics' association with mortality or cancer: a matched cohort study.' *British Medical Journal Open*, 2012; 2:e000850 DOI: 10.1136/bmjopen-2012-00085

Chapter 11

1. Lazarus, R, Folkman, S. *Stress, Appraisal, and Coping*, (New York: Springer Publishing, 1984)

2. Epel, ES, Lin, J, Dhabhar FS, Wolkowitz, OM, et al. 'Dynamics of telomerase activity in response to acute psychological stress.' *Brain, Behavior, and Immunity*, 2010 May, 24 (4): 531–539. Doi:10.1016/j. bbi.2009.11.018. PMC 2856774. PMID 20018236

3. Irwin, M. 'Psychoneuroimmunology of depression: clinical implications.' *Brain, Behavior, and Immunity*, 2002, 16, 1–16

4. Eremin, O. 'Immuno-modulatory effects of relaxation training and guided imagery in women with locally advanced breast cancer undergoing multimodality therapy: a randomised controlled trial.' *The Breast* 18, 2009, 17–25.

5. Courtney R, Cohen M, Van Dixhoorn J. 'Relationship between dysfunctional breathing patterns and ability to achieve target heart rate variability with features of "coherence" during biofeedback.' *Alternatives to Therapies in Health and Medicine*. May–June 2011, 17(3): 38–44

6. Mental Health Foundation: Up and Running? Report. March 2005

7. World Health Organization; Global Recommendations on Physical Activity for Health, http://www.who.int/dietphysicalactivity/factsheet_adults/en

8. http://www.simplydivinerelationshiptraining.com

9. www.emofree.com

10. http://www.sciencedaily.com/releases/2011/03/110301122156.htm

11. Bennett, M and Lengacher, C. 'Humor and Laughter May Influence Health: III. Laughter and Health Outcomes, Indiana State University College of Nursing and University of South Florida.' eCAM 2008; 5 (1) 37–40

12. Umberson, D and Montez, JK. 'Social Relationships and Health: A Flashpoint for Health Policy.' *Journal of Health and Social Behaviour*, 2010; 51. http://www.ncbi.nlm.nih.gov/pmc/articles/PMC3150158/

13. Robbins, John. *Healthy at 100: The Scientifically Proven Secrets of the World's Healthiest and Longest-Lived Peoples*, (New York: Ballantine Books, 2008)

CHAPTER 12

1. 'High dose vitamin and mineral supplements in the UK.' Food Standard Agency, December 2006. http://www.food.gov.uk/science/research/surveillance/fsisbranch2006/fsis1206#.Us3IqBaCbzI

2. Scheer, Roddy and Moss, Doug. 'Dirt poor: have fruit and vegetables become less nutritious?' *Scientific American, Energy and Sustainability Issue*. April 2011

3. Grodstein, F, et al. 'Long-term multivitamin supplementation and cognitive function in men: a randomized trial.' *Annals of Internal Medicine.* Dec 2013, 159(12): 806–814

4. Lamas, G, et al. 'Oral high-dose multivitamins and minerals after myocardial infarction: a randomized trial.' *Annals of Internal Medicine.* Dec 2013, 159 (12): 797–805

5. Fortmann, S, et al. 'Vitamin and mineral supplements in the primary prevention of cardiovascular disease and cancer: an updated systematic evidence review for the US Preventative Services Task Force.' *Annals of Internal Medicine,* Dec 2013, 159 (12): 824–834

6. Michels, Alexander and Frei, Balz. 'Myths, artifacts, and fatal flaws: identifying limitations and opportunities in vitamin C research.' *Nutrients,* 2013; 5 (12): 5161

7. Brasky, TM, et al. 'Plasma phospholipid fatty acids and prostate cancer risk in the SELECT trial.' *Journal of The National Cancer Institute,* August 2013

8. Szymanski, KM, et al. 'Fish consumption and prostate cancer risk: a review and meta-analysis.' *American Journal of Clinical Nutrition,* Nov 2010; 92(5): 1223–33

9. Rundle, A, et al. 'Obesity and future prostate cancer risk among men after an initial benign biopsy of the prostate.' *Cancer Epidemiology, Biomarkers and Prevention,* April 2013

10. Barton, DL, et al. Pilot study of Panax quinquefolius (American ginseng) to improve cancer-related fatigue: a randomized, double-blind dose-finding evaluation. *Support Care Cancer,* Feb 2010, 8(2):179–87

Chapter 14

With thanks to Dr Marion Gluck at The Marion Gluck Clinic – www.mariongluckclinic.com

1. Women's Health Initiative Study 2002 – http://www.nhlbi.nih.gov/news/press-releases/2002/nhlbi-stops-trial-of-estrogen-plus-progestin-due-to-increased-breast-cancer-risk-lack-of-overall-benefit.html

2. Wang, C, et al. 'Low testosterone associated with obesity and the metabolic syndrome contributes to sexual dysfunction and cardiovascular disease risk in men with type 2 diabetes.' *Diabetes Care,* Jul 2011 vol. 34 no. 7 1669–1675

RESOURCES

FURTHER READING

Atkinson, Mark. *The Mind–Body Bible*, (London: Piatkus, 2007)

Barnouin K, Freedman, R. *Skinny Bitch*, (Philadelphia: Running Press, 2005)

Carr, Kris. *Crazy Sexy Diet: Eat Your Veggies, Ignite Your Spark, and Live Like You Mean It!*, (Connecticut, Skirt!, 2011)

Corrett, N, and Edgson, V. *Honestly Healthy: Eat with your body in mind, the alkaline way*, (London, Jacqui Small LLP, 2012)

Gluck, M, Dr and Edgson, V. *It Must Be My Hormones*, (London: Penguin, 2010)

Junger, Alejandro. *Clean: The Revolutionary Program to Restore the Body's Natural Ability to Heal Itself*, (London, HarperOne, 2012)

Lipman, Frank. *Revive!: End Exhaustion & Feel Great Again*, (London, Hay House, 2012)

Moritz, Andreas. *The Liver and Gallbladder Mirlcle cleanse*, (Berkeley: Ulysees Prers, 2009)

Ornish, Dean. *The Spectrum: A Scientifically Proven Program to Feel Better, Live Longer, Lose Weight and Gain Health*, (New York: Ballantine Books, 2007)

Penman, D, Dr and Williams, M Prof. *Mindfulness: A Practical Guide to Finding Peace in a Frantic World*, (London: Little, Brown, 2011)

Pinnock, D. *The Medicinal Chef: Eat Your Way to Better Health* (London, Quadrille Publishing Ltd, 2013)

Reiss, Uzzi. *The Natural Superwoman: The Scientifically Backed Program for Feeling Great, Looking Younger, and Enjoying Amazing Energy at Any Age*, (New York, Avery Publishing Group, 2008)

Robbins, John. *Healthy at 100: The Scientifically Proven Secrets of the World's Healthiest and Longest-Lived Peoples*, (New York, Ballantine Books, 2008)

Somers, Suzanne, *I'm Too Young for This!: The Natural Hormone Solution to Enjoy Perimenopause*, (New York, Harmony, 2013)

SUPPLEMENTS – REPUTABLE SOURCES I REGULARLY USE

Bionutri Supplements – www.bionutri.co.uk. I regularly use Ecodophilus, Ecobalance and Ecogest to heal leaky gut syndrome and aid removal of candida

Higher Nature – www.highernature.co.uk. Higher nature make good quality supplements and their range spans from multivitamins to specific supplements that can help support hair and skin, bone health and the immune system to name but a few.

Nutri Supplements – www.nutri-online1.co.uk. Nutri are a brand that produce high quality supplements and are also committed to teaching and training practitioners. They produce 'medical meal replacement' shakes, supplements to support the adrenal glands and good quality vitamin, mineral and fish oil supplements.

Planet Health – http://uk.planethealth.com.au for good-quality spirulina and other supplements in their lifestream range

Revital – www.revital.co.uk stock a good variety and quality of supplements

Spatone – a milder iron supplement with less gastrointestinal side effects

DIAGNOSTIC TESTS

Genova Diagnostics – www.gdx.net and nelsonsnaturalworld.com can carry out tests for candida, leaky gut, parasites and bacteria in the bowel and adrenal fatigue

YOGA AND MINDFULNESS

Brown, Christine. *The Yoga Bible*, (London, Godsfield Press, 2009)

Fraser, Tara. *The Easy Yoga Workout*, (London, Watkins Publishing LTD, 2010)

Headspace – www.getsomeheadspace.com a free daily meditation app

Kabat-Zinn, John. *Guided Mindfulness Meditation*, audio CD, (Louisville, Sounds True Inc, 2005)

Maya Fiennes: www.mayaspace.com

Simply Yoga – a free app that has 20, 40 and 60 minute workouts that you can follow on your android phone or tablet

The British Wheel of Yoga – www.bwy.org.uk a resource to learn about yoga and search for teachers in the UK

Yoga Journal – www.yogajournal.com an online resource that goes through various poses and sequences

ACKNOWLEDGEMENTS

I'm extremely lucky to have an incredible support network of family and friends and colleagues. My sister Zairah, I'm glad we have become such good friends as we've got older, and I finally have a brother in Stephen.

I have such lovely friends, they are truly the 'family I've chosen for myself'. Temi Odetoyinbo, Martin Edwards, Gareth Cooze-Rees – you are my rocks, I love you. Thank you for everything you do for me and for putting up with me when I am being hard work! My other nearest and dearest who have supported me through the birth of this book are the REPC/Fight Club crew, Sarah Lane, Lindsay Millward, Lucy James, Ian Collings and Tony Munoz, as well as Angela Dwyer for being with me the day I discovered integrative medicine and chose my path. To all my other friends I haven't been able to mention, it doesn't mean I love you any less and am grateful that you are in my life.

My business pals Cheryl Bass from I AM WOMAN, Kathryn Rogers, Radha Vyas, Sheilagh Blyth, Sara Tye and all at redheadPR and especially Elizabeth Inniss who has supported me every step of the book-writing process.

In terms of people who have helped me in my journey in integrative medicine – Dr Mark Atkinson was the inspiration whose book led me to integrative medicine. I've had some great mentors but special thanks goes to Dr Rosy Daniel, Dr Wendy Denning and Dr Marion Gluck and all the team at The Marion Gluck Clinic. Also thanks to my GP mentors Dr Rob Morgan and Dr Huw Mason.

Thanks to Fiona Harrold, Sam Jackson and Justine Taylor, and all at Ebury Publishing for allowing me to have this wonderful opportunity to spread my message.

Finally, thank you to Russell Brand and Noel Gallagher for making me smile and boosting my energy reserves when I need it, your work has inspired me more than you'll ever know.

INDEX